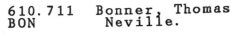
MAR – – 1993

| DATE | | | |
|---|---|---|---|
| | | | |
| | | | |
| | | | |
| | | | |
| | | | |
| | | | |
| | | | |
| | | | |
| | | | |
| | | | |
| | | | |
| | | | |
| | | | |

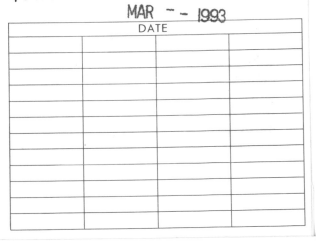

*To the Ends of the Earth*

# To the Ends of the Earth

*Women's Search for Education in Medicine*

Thomas Neville Bonner

Harvard University Press
Cambridge, Massachusetts
London, England
1992

*Library of Congress Cataloging-in-Publication Data*

Bonner, Thomas Neville.
    To the ends of the earth : women's search for education in
  medicine / Thomas Neville Bonner.
        p.   cm.
  Includes bibliographical references and index.
  ISBN 0-674-89303-4 (alk. paper)
    1. Women in medicine—History.   2. Women medical students—
  History.   I. Title.
  [DNLM: 1. Education, Medical—history.   2. Physicians, Women—
  history.   W 18 B716t]
  R692.B66   1992
  610'.71'1—dc20
  DNLM/DLC                        91-20826
  for Library of Congress              CIP

For Sylvia
Die alles ermöglicht

# Preface

Over thirty years ago, while doing research on American doctors in European universities before 1914, I came upon the remarkable number of foreign women, including Americans, who were enrolled in medicine at Zurich, Bern, Paris, and Geneva. Although my primary interest was in postgraduate study, largely by men, I could not help noticing the strong impact that these women enrolled in medical courses had on academic and political life in every university town where they were found.

What were they doing there? Why should American women be learning medicine in Zurich or Paris or Geneva in 1870 or 1895? What drove hundreds, at times thousands, of Russian and East European women west to Swiss or French medical schools for half a century? Why were so many English women to be found in Paris or Brussels, and so many German women in Zurich and Bern? What must conditions have been like in their homelands to propel so many to study in foreign lands hundreds or thousands of miles distant from their homes and families? What drove them to forsake familiar surroundings, their native tongues, and established expectations and to exile themselves abroad?

The more I asked such questions, the greater my curiosity. Little had been written, I quickly found, about women's search for medical training, either at home or abroad, in the half-century before Sarajevo. Much of what has since been published is from the perspective of a single country and misses the international dimension of the medical women's movement. For in every major country women were seeking in these years, in different ways and with differing success, to qualify themselves to practice medicine. Their stubborn striving to enter a male-dominated profession grew out of sweeping economic and cultural changes in their own lives that coincided with powerful changes in higher education and medicine itself. These were critical years in the Western world for university reform, new ideas about women, a rising faith in science, and efforts to control access to the learned professions. Against the backdrop of new images of science and old sexual stereotypes, the women of many countries fought to establish a niche for themselves in the emerging profession of scientific medicine.

But the women of different nations were affected in different ways by the forces of change. Women in the United States, benefiting from the loose, laissez-faire, private structures of American society, were early able to establish separate schools of medicine and separate hospitals when the established institutions refused them, but these same structures made possible stiff resistance later to breaking down remaining sexual barriers to medical assimilation. British and Canadian women, faced with a similarly unflinching resistance to co-education, likewise depended on privately supported hospitals and medical schools for women as the principal route to medical learning throughout the nineteenth and early twentieth centuries.

The independent-minded Swiss, on the other hand, were the first to open their medical schools fully to women by state action, to be followed by the French and then most of the smaller nations of the European continent. In Tsarist Russia, a complex and divided governing class, challenged constantly by intellectuals and academic authorities, alternated between barring women completely from medical study and allowing a limited number of them into special women's courses. Imperial Germany, the most fiercely resistant of all to the idea of women doctors, capitulated altogether in 1908 and was soon educating more women physicians than even the United States. Outside Europe and North America, such major nations as India, China, and Japan followed European patterns in bringing women into medicine, either by barring women altogether from medical study, by founding separate women's schools, or by allowing women to go abroad to study.

# Acknowledgments

The debts I have gathered in completing this work are unusually large. For a summer of investigation of materials in Switzerland and Paris in 1986 I am indebted to the American Philosophical Society for a timely grant. An appointment as Visiting Historical Scholar at the National Library of Medicine in 1987 enabled me to do further background reading on the subject. Wayne State University supported research visits to important repositories in Boston, Northampton, Philadelphia, and Germany.

A large vote of thanks is due to the many librarians, archivists, and scholars who have helped me in my researches. I want above all to thank Huldrych M. Koelbing and his staff, especially Frau Seger, at the Medizinhistorisches Institut of the University of Zurich for their many kindnesses. Others who helped in important ways were Urs Boschung, Ulrich Im Hof, Ladislaw Myzyrowicz, Jean Starobinski, and Werner G. Zimmermann, all of Switzerland; Johanna Bleker, Mariella Böhme, G. Fichtner, Hans H. Lauer, Helmut Leitner, and H. Schott of Germany; Mary Ann Elston, England; Rose Sheinen, Canada; and Selma Calmes, Linda Goldstein, and Todd L. Savitt of the United States. Among many helpful librarians and archivists, I am especially grateful to Margaret Jerrido of the Archives and Special Collections on Women in Medicine at the Medical College of Pennsylvania, Susan Boone of the Sophia Smith Collection, Smith College, the several helpful archivists at the Schlesinger Library, Radcliffe College, Richard J. Wolfe of the Francis A. Countway Library of Medicine, Harvard Medical School, and, most important of all, Ruth Taylor and her colleagues of the Wayne State University Libraries.

Several scholars have been generous in reading portions or all of the manuscript and making suggestions. I want to express my gratitude to Pamela Sears McKinsey, James Albisetti, Guy Stern, Mary Ann Elston, Johanna Bleker, and Donna Evleth, for reading and commenting on one or more chapters. Others who read the entire manuscript conscientiously are Regina M. Morantz-Sanchez and Ellen More. To all of them I am deeply grateful. A special appreciation is due also to Monika Bankowski of the Center for Slavic Studies, University of Zurich, for her many kindnesses in running down references, sending me materials, and critically reading Chapters 2–4. All of these colleagues have saved me from errors of fact and interpretation, but doubtless others remain to become my responsibility.

Appreciation is due to the *Bulletin of the History of Medicine* and the *Journal of the History of Medicine and Allied Sciences* for allowing me to use portions of articles that appeared earlier in these journals.

The translations from German and French in the text are my own, those from Russian are the work of Pamela Sears McKinsey.

I want finally to thank Ginny Corbin for an unusually conscientious and patient typing and retyping of the manuscript, and John Stewart for his invaluable help in preparing the index.

# Contents

# Illustrations

*To the Ends of the Earth*

If you were a young man, I could not find words in which to express my satisfaction and pride in respect to your [medical career] . . . but you are a woman, a weak woman; and all that I can do for you is to grieve and to weep. O my daughter! return from this unhappy path.

Letter to Marie E. Zakrzewska, M.D.,<br>from her father, 1855

If I were to plan with malicious hate the greatest curse I could conceive for woman, if I would estrange them from the protection of woman, and make them as far as possible loathsome and disgusting to man, I would favor the so-called reform which proposed to make doctors of them.

*Buffalo Medical Journal*, 1869

I think only the university is worth so much that a woman could sacrifice all for it. Only it is worth visiting notwithstanding scant means or other inconveniences. But in Russia this way is closed to woman, because for her the doors of the university are closed like those of the altar . . . I shall stop at nothing, because this whole plan [to go to Zurich] is not the product of idle fantasy, but my flesh and blood.

Vera Figner, 1872

At what sacrifice have [women] struggled to obtain the elusive prize! They have starved on half rations, shivered in cold rooms . . . when they were not permitted to walk, they have crept,—where they could not take, they have begged; they have gleaned like Ruth among the harvesters for the scantiest crumbs of knowledge, and been thankful.

Mary Putnam Jacobi, 1891

# *Prologue: 1871*

Paris, midsummer, 1871. The long siege of the city by Prussian troops was ended. Everywhere there was a feeling of relief after the months of suffering, hunger, and cold. Gradually, life returned to normal in the defeated capital. The victorious Prussians had remained as occupiers, however, as they proclaimed a new German Empire in the great palace at Versailles. In France and throughout Europe came a vivid sense of old foundations crumbling and a new and uncertain future in the making.

In Paris, the venerable Ecole de Médecine had reopened as professors and students alike returned from war service to their studies. Many of them had served in medical units at Sedan, Belfort, Metz, or Strasbourg. Among the civilian students finishing their studies that summer was a young American woman. Twenty-nine years old, Mary Corinna Putnam, daughter of the New York publisher G. P. Putnam, had been in Paris for five years. Her French fiancé had just returned from military duty, but she found him changed and the relationship cooled. Gradually, she had overcome obstacle after obstacle to gain the right to enter special lectures, clinics, and the ancient library of medicine. With the help of the minister of education, she had been able to circumvent the opposition of a hostile faculty and to enroll at last in an official course of lectures. In the lectures, in deference to male sensitivities, she was required to sit in a separate chair near the lectern and to enter the hall through a side door. It was all a practical stratagem, she told her mother, to outflank the faculty "by an adroit maneuver." Finally, in 1868, she had become the first woman ever to matriculate in the school of medicine.[1]

On 24 July 1871, she stood before the formally attired members of the Paris faculty to defend her thesis on "La Graisse neutres et les acides gras" (Fats and Fatty Acids). Those present recalled especially her small stature, her dark, tightly drawn hair, and her confident manner. She reminded some of a serious, no-nonsense school-teacher. A band of three hundred curious students and physicians had crowded into the ascending tiers of the auditorium. With more than a touch of irony, she had dedicated her thesis, according to the Archives de Médecine, "To the professor, whose name I do not know, who was the only one to vote for my admission to the school, thus protesting against the prejudice which would exclude women from advanced studies."[2] The questioning by the professors, by all accounts, was probing but friendly. When the examination was over, she was asked to leave the room while her performance was judged. On her return, she was congratulated warmly by her examiners, while the audience, some of them standing, applauded. Her defense of her thesis, as described in faculty records, was judged to be *extrêmement satisfait*.[3] The faculty awarded her a bronze medal for her work, one of only three such awards to go to women in the first twenty years of women's study in Paris.[4]

Putnam was not the only American woman finishing a European medical degree that eventful year. Three hundred sixty miles to the southeast and three months later, Susan Dimock of North Carolina followed another academic procession into the examination room at the University of Zurich. Leading the procession was the rector of the university, closely followed by the colorfully robed members of the medical faculty, with Dimock at the rear. She took her place next to the rector at the head of the long, narrow table, which was draped for the occasion with a green felt cloth. As in Paris, dozens of curious students and physicians had come to see and hear the young American. She was twenty-four years old, serious, thoughtful, and attractive in appearance. She was questioned at length by her professors and by members of the audience on her dissertation concerning "The Different Forms of Puerperal Fever." When they were finished, the anatomist Hermann von Meyer, a friend of women's education, rose to tell her: "You have shown by your example that it is possible for women to devote themselves to the medical profession without denying your female nature."[5] From Zurich, she would travel to Vienna, where a woman physician was an even greater rarity than in Zurich. One of her clinical teachers there would later write: "The question, whether a woman can be fit for the study and practice of medicine, has been definitely answered by the appearance of Dr. Susan Dimock."[6]

Dimock and Putnam were thus the first Americans to join a growing procession of young women from many countries who were driven into self-imposed exile by their ambition to qualify themselves as thoroughly as men to practice medicine. They were extraordinary, not only because they were the first women from the United States to complete a medical degree in Europe, but also because they were among the first women from any country to complete the rigorous training for a European medical degree.

Both women had grown up in the rapidly changing era preceding the Civil War in America. The lives of both had been touched by the growing women's movement of the past quarter-century. Like many of the pioneer women in medicine, they had spent their formative years in comfortable middle-class families headed by professional men with progressive views about women. Both had shown determination early to make a career in a profession known for its inhospitability to women. Both had served as interns in the women-run New England Hospital for Women and Children. And both were determined to find a kind of medical education not then possible for women in the special hospitals and medical schools for women throughout the United States. Putnam, in fact, had already earned a degree at the Woman's Medical College of Pennsylvania.

Now, in 1871, they had won European degrees after completing the most comprehensive medical training open to women in the nineteenth century. For Europe, and especially Paris and the German-speaking universities of Austria, Switzerland, and Germany itself, was the mecca in these years for all those Americans who wanted to learn the best in modern medicine. Thousands of Americans went to Berlin or Zurich or Paris to learn what they could not learn in Cambridge or Philadelphia or Chicago.

For a time, Paris and Zurich were the only cities in the world where women could learn scientific medicine on the same basis as men. The Paris correspondent of the *New York Tribune*, who had followed Putnam's trials and been present at one of her qualifying examinations, chided Americans for forcing women to take a "weak, flavorless, uninspiriting course of second hand lectures delivered by

an unwilling professor to women alone." He contrasted the attitude
and behavior of French students and professors with the recent coarse
and hostile reception given women students by their male colleagues
in Philadelphia. "This is the way, oh boys of Philadelphia," he concluded a description of the treatment given Mary Putnam, "that
women are treated in the greatest University in the world."[7]

The "boys of Philadelphia" were not different, of course, from the
boys of New York and Chicago in 1871, or for that matter from those
of Edinburgh and Berlin, in their contempt and derision of those few
women who ventured to study medicine. At the Pennsylvania Hospital, at about the time of the examination described by the Paris
correspondent, the students had greeted the first women allowed
into its clinics, according to an eyewitness, with "insolent and offensive language . . . missiles of paper, tin foil, tobacco-quids, etc. . . .
while some of these men defiled the dresses of the ladies near them
with tobacco juice."[8] A student who sat through the clinics had
written in her diary of "the groans and hisses of as *ungentlemanly* a
set of fellows as one would care to meet."[9] In Chicago, students at
the Chicago Medical College had made life likewise unpleasant for
the first women students in 1870 and demanded their expulsion,
claiming that because of their presence "certain materials and observations have been omitted."[10] The students were only following
the example of their teachers. No American medical college, with
the exception of women's and sectarian schools, freely admitted
women before 1870. The leading medical men of New York, Boston,
Philadelphia, and Chicago were nearly unanimous in their hostility
to educating women in medicine, especially in mixed classes. Nathan
Smith Davis, for example, the influential founder of the American
Medical Association, spoke for many when he told his Chicago colleagues in 1869, when the question of women doctors came up, that
"to appropriately fill this exalted position [of being mother to the
race] is job enough for any woman."[11]

Yet, by the time Davis spoke, the United States was educating
more women doctors than the rest of the world combined. A total
of 525 women physicians were counted in the census of 1870.[12]
From all corners of the globe came queries about America's success
in overcoming ancient prejudices and modern strictures against
women's medical study.

What had happened? How was it that the United States, in spite
of the hostile attitudes of male physicians and educators, was able

for several decades to outdistance Europe and the world in teaching medicine to women? Where did they study? How were they prepared? Why did Europeans, in general, not follow the American example? And why did Mary Putnam and Susan Dimock feel it necessary to go to Paris and Zurich to learn medicine? These are some of the questions to be taken up in the following pages.

# 1 *Women and the Study of Medicine*

The path to a medical degree for a woman, strewn with obstacles as it was in 1871, was incomparably smoother than it had been twenty years before. In all the world in 1850, no regularly established medical school anywhere consistently opened its doors to women. The Geneva Medical College in rural New York, which had gained worldwide fame for allowing Elizabeth Blackwell to enter in 1847, had hastily slammed its doors shut after she graduated. "Miss Blackwell's admission was an *experiment,* not intended as a *precedent,*" insisted Dean James Hadley in 1849 to a second applicant, Sarah R. Adamson, who had already been turned down by three colleges in Philadelphia.[1] The experiment, by the dean's accounting, had been a failure. In Cleveland, another woman, Nancy Talbot Clark, managed to be admitted to the medical department of the Western Reserve College, thanks to the dean and a sympathetic faculty member, in 1851 and was followed by five other women in the next few years before that school, too, changed its mind and barred entrance to further women.[2] Farther west, Elizabeth Blackwell's sister Emily was able to enroll for a term at the Rush Medical College in Chicago but was then, in the wake of student and professional protests, denied the right to complete her degree. She became one of the six women to find refuge in Cleveland. The Chicago school was promptly censured by the state medical society for its "impropriety in admitting a woman."[3]

Everywhere, the story was the same. When Sarah Adamson applied to the Jefferson Medical College in Philadelphia, the dean told her that "it would be impossible in this country for a lady to mingle with five hundred young men . . . in the same lecture room, without experiencing many annoyances."⁴ At Harvard, Harriot Hunt, who had been practicing medicine in Boston without formal training for a dozen years, almost gained entry to the famous medical school in 1850 before finally being told that "the faculty feared the students would leave Harvard and go to Yale upon the advent of a woman student."⁵ Given student attitudes in places such as Harvard, the faculty may well have been right. The Harvard students, in any case, explained their opposition to women colleagues forthrightly in a series of public resolutions:⁶

> *Resolved,* that no woman of true delicacy would be willing in the presence of men to listen to the discussion of the subjects that necessarily come under the consideration of the student of medicine.
>
> *Resolved,* that we object to having the company of any female forced upon us, who is disposed to unsex herself, and to sacrifice her modesty, by appearing with men in the medical lecture room.

Small wonder then that few women braved the censure and ridicule of their contemporaries to seek a problematic career in medicine. "There was not a woman physician in any city," said the German immigrant Marie Zakrzewska of her arrival in 1853, "who could support herself from the result of her studies . . ." The status of the handful of women physicians of that era she described as "pitiable, ignominious, and despised." None of the pioneer women doctors of the 1850s was well prepared for her tasks, since their male teachers "did not dare introduce them, as they did their male students, into the houses of even their poorest patients and give them the opportunity for practical knowledge."⁷ The derision faced by the first graduates was universal. When Hannah Longshore first began to practice medicine in Philadelphia in 1851, for example, a leading pharmacist refused at first to sell her drugs, telling her: "You are out of your sphere! Go home and darn your husband's stockings! Housekeeping is the business for women."⁸

The ban against women's study in 1850 was even more stringent in the great medical centers of Europe. The name of not a single medical woman appears in the British Medical Directory of that year. For another quarter-century, the efforts of British women to gain a place in medicine were systematically resisted or crushed. Only Elizabeth Blackwell, educated in America, and Elizabeth Garrett, who won an apothecary's license before the rules were changed to bar women, were officially recognized as practitioners of medicine in Britain before 1877.[9] In France, no woman was allowed to register for medical study until Mary Putnam was admitted in 1868, and few French women were able to meet the educational requirements thereafter. Virtually nowhere in Europe were women admitted to the strenuous secondary schools that alone could qualify a student for admission to the university.[10] Although the Italian universities historically had been open to women, the first modern woman to matriculate in medicine did not do so until 1876.[11] Austria barred women from entering medical schools until the end of the century and kept them out of law schools until the First World War.[12] In Germany, the center of enlightened medical science after 1870, women were officially banned from medical study until 1900; in Prussia, until 1908. Even then, the Prussian law permitted individual faculty members to prohibit women from attending their lectures.[13]

## Women in an Economic Squeeze

Across the Western world, the position of the nineteenth-century woman in industrial society was in crisis. A social revolution was transforming the traditional relationships of women to the family and to the world of work. In England and America especially the industrial changes were creating a chasm between the new class of working women and the sheltered daughters of the middle class.[14] The economic transformation of Europe since the end of the eighteenth century, together with the liberating ideas unloosed by the French Revolution, had made the "woman question" a subject of intense political and social interest in nearly every country. Particularly in the ascendant middle classes was the new diminished productive role of women within the family a source of anxious concern. To many in the rising merchant and professional elite, it became a matter of pride that wives and daughters had no need to work. Women were now seen as guardians of older values in the new era of harsh competition and worker exploitation. As Sara Evans has written:

> If men were competitive, women exemplified cooperation; if men could reason, women were emotional and irrational; if men were building

an increasingly secular and amoral political and economic order, women sustained piety and morality; if men sought dominance, women would submit; if men occupied the public sphere, women ruled in their own private, domestic realm, the home.[15]

A biological view of women that paralleled their lessened social role grew up in medical and scientific circles. The qualities so highly valued in women by Victorian society—gentility, spirituality, and moral strength—were now assumed to be related to women's weaker physical constitution. A woman was smaller of stature, she lacked muscular strength, her brain capacity was less than a man's, and her nervous system was far more delicate than that of men. She was furthermore always at the mercy of her reproductive organs, which made her behavior emotional, erratic, and unpredictable.[16] "One-fourth of the active period of a woman's life," the surgeon D. Hayes Agnew told his students at the University of Pennsylvania in 1870, "she is under the perturbating influence of a function . . . in which neither the mind nor body are in a condition to meet the demands of a profession."[17]

The Victorian reaction to women doctors was one of shock and disbelief. The presence of a woman in a hospital, a clinic, or, even worse, a lecture on male anatomy or women's diseases, violated every precept of society's code for the conduct of females. The division of roles between men and women in polite society made it unthinkable for one to step over the boundary into the other's preserve. "Woman was obviously designed to move in another sphere, to discharge other duties," declared the editor of the *Boston Medical and Surgical Journal* in 1849, in denouncing Elizabeth Blackwell's graduation as a "farce." Her duties were

> not less important, not less honorable, but more refined, more delicate. Within her province she is all powerful. She is the pride and glory of the race—the sacred repository of all that is virtuous and graceful and lovely. But when she departs from this, she goes astray from her appropriate element, dishonors her sex, seeks laurels in forbidden paths, and perverts the laws of her Maker.[18]

Woman's biological nature and her role in society made necessary a special kind of education. "The idealized weakness of women, their pliable nature . . . and their capacity to acquiesce and still take care of husband and child," writes Johanna Geyer-Kordesch, "were impregnated early and carried over to girls' education."[19] Women themselves internalized much of the biological determinism of the era. The young middle-class woman of the 1850s in Europe and America was brought up for a lifelong career as wife and mother. She learned little beyond the basic skills needed for communication and understanding her religion and perhaps some private instruction in sketching, embroidery, or music. Science, mathematics, and classical studies were rarely a part of her upbringing.[20] A European woman was strictly segregated from young men in school and could not be admitted to a gymnasium or a lycée that prepared students for the university.[21] While coeducation was more common in England and America, it did not extend to the private academy in the United States or to the English public school. To a growing number of women and their liberal supporters, the reform of education was more and more seen as the first critical step to economic opportunity and social independence for women outside the diminished family. For the pioneer generation of women doctors especially, the struggle to gain a general scientific education outside the male-dominated school system was often as fierce as the battle to get an education in medicine itself.

## Why Women Should Not Be Doctors

The quest for higher learning by women raised special questions in the case of medicine. Did women possess the intellectual capacity necessary to master a learned profession? Were they hardy enough to carry on a medical and surgical practice? Were pregnancy and menstruation not insuperable barriers to a profession in which constant attention to duty was an indispensable requirement? Would the study of anatomy and dissection of the human body not destroy the special sensibilities of women? Would not their presence in mixed classes inhibit the medical professors from free discussion of sensitive subjects and keep medical students from raising questions that might be embarrassing to women? For three-quarters of a century, these all-too-familiar questions were raised over and over again in debates that raged from Moscow to San Francisco, and from Oslo to Cape-town. Less frequently heard was the concern of physicians in many countries about heightened economic competition from women in a profession that was already suffering from overcrowding and low public esteem.

The opposition to women doctors was overwhelming in Europe and only slightly less hostile in America. In Germany, the renowned Munich anatomist Theodor von Bischoff summed up a generation's thinking in 1872 when he argued that woman's smaller brain, her physical weakness, and her gentle nature unfitted her for medical science. "Medical study," he charged in a fifty-six-page pamphlet that became the Bible of opponents of women's study, "contradicts and hurts the best and most noble side of feminine nature." By both the divine and the natural order, women lacked the rare ability to work in the natural sciences and especially medicine.[22] The German-born Marie Zakrzewska recalled with sorrow a letter she received from her father lamenting her unfortunate choice of career. "If you were a young man," he wrote, "I could not find words in which to express my satisfaction and pride in respect to your acts . . . but you are a woman, a weak woman; and all that I can do for you now is to grieve and to weep. O my daughter! return from this unhappy path."[23] In Great Britain, physicians and public alike decried the efforts of young women to gain entrance to medicine. Professor Thomas Laycock of the University of Edinburgh spoke for many in 1869 when he told Sophia Jex-Blake flatly that he "could not imagine *any decent woman* wishing to study medicine;—as for any *lady*, that was out of the question."[24] And the father of young Elizabeth Garrett, upon being told that his beloved daughter wanted to become a doctor, burst out: "The whole idea is so *disgusting*. I could not entertain it for a moment."[25]

Attitudes in France were hardly different from those of Germany and Britain until at least the 1870s. Although women were not excluded by law from the professions or from higher education after 1863, they were rarely able to get the secondary school preparation needed to apply for admission to the universities.[26] Elizabeth Blackwell, who had gone to Paris for clinical experience, described her term at La Maternité hospital in Paris as her "prison life" and told her mother that French physicians "are determined not to grant the slightest favour to a feminine M.D."[27] She was treated, despite her medical degree, like a midwife-in-training, enduring a regimen of communal living, frequent night duty, constant menial assignments, and "virtual imprisonment on the grounds of the hospital."[28] The difference in hostility between French and English opponents of women studying medicine, Mary Putnam wrote in her witty style, was that

> An Englishman would say that it was indelicate to admit women to study medicine, a Frenchman, that it was dangerous. The French disbelief in women is so rooted, and their whole social system is constructed so entirely on the principle of keeping young men and women as far apart as flame and gunpowder, that they would consider as a perfect absurdity any attempt on the part of their own countrywomen to study medicine . . . I suppose that I am considered very much of an anomaly, but the peculiarity is attributed to the influence of Americanism.[29]

The few American women who had been able to enter the profession before 1860 faced further barriers once they sought to begin a practice. As Richard Shryock has written, American women encountered multiple layers of conservative defense: if women were somehow able to enter a medical school, the hospitals were closed to them; if hospital experience was permitted, then internship opportunities were denied; and later, in many places, they would be virtually banned from consulting with experienced male practitioners.[30] American parents and the public generally shared the European disdain for a woman entering medicine. The mother of Eliza Mosher, an early medical graduate of the University of Michigan, told her that she would rather see her in a mental asylum than in the practice of medicine.[31] Mary Putnam's father likewise thought medicine a "repulsive pursuit" for a woman.[32] A male physician friend of Marie Zakrzewska's wrote her in 1860: "I have put it to myself whether I could be willing that one of my daughters should go through the discipline and lead the life that I have done myself. The idea is intolerable."[33] Once she graduated from medical school, Zakrzewska, like other pioneers, found it impossible to rent rooms for medical practice, and was forced to take Elizabeth Blackwell's back parlor in New York.[34] Blackwell herself suffered from malicious gossip and unwanted attentions from New York men. "I understand now," she wrote, "why this life has never been lived before. It *is* hard, with no support but a high purpose, to live against every species of social opposition . . . I *should* like a little fun now and then. Life is altogether too sober."[35]

## The American Context

How was it, then, that American women, despite the overwhelming opposition of the medical profession and much of the public, were able to practice medicine for a time in much larger numbers than their sisters across the Atlantic? Even in neighboring Canada, no woman was allowed to enter a medical school until the 1880s. But women doctors were appearing in community after community across the United States in the 1850s. Harriot Hunt, long the only woman practicing in Boston, was joined in the early 1850s by two women physicians, Nancy Talbot Clark, the first woman to graduate from the Western Reserve College in Cleveland, and Martha Sawin, a member of the first graduating class of the new medical college for women in Philadelphia.[36] Two of Clark's sister graduates in Cleveland, Emily Blackwell and Marie Zakrzewska, meanwhile joined Elizabeth Blackwell in practice in New York. In Philadelphia, many of those who won degrees at the Woman's Medical College of Pennsylvania, or at the eclectic Penn Medical University, stayed in the city to begin their medical work. The latter school, particularly frowned upon by the regular profession, had graduated more women by 1864 than any other medical school in the country.[37]

There were other early centers of women physicians. In western New York, the Nantucket-born Lydia Folger Fowler won a degree at the short-lived Eclectic Medical College, then located in Rochester, later in Syracuse, and became the first woman to teach medical students when she was given a teaching position in that school. Thirteen other women, including Sarah Adamson Dolley, Rachel Brooks Gleason, and the Civil War surgeon Mary Walker, took classes at the school in Rochester or in Syracuse.[38] Another of the school's graduates, the health reformer Clemence Lozier, founded a homeopathic college for women in New York in 1863, which would enroll close to a hundred students in its first seven years.[39] Farther west, Harriot Hunt discovered ten women studying medicine in Cincinnati in 1855 at an eclectic medical college.[40] In Cleveland, a homeopathic college launched in 1850 allowed three women into its first class and succeeded in graduating twelve women by 1860. On the west coast, Toland Medical College in San Francisco counted a lone woman in its first graduating class in 1864.[41]

As early as 1859, Elizabeth Blackwell estimated that three hundred American women had managed, in her words, "to graduate somewhere in medicine."[42] More recently, Professor Edward Atwater has counted 247 women graduates as of the beginning of the Civil War.[43] Those practicing, it has long been known, included adherents of the informal botanic schools, which had flourished in the years before 1850. Of the more than five hundred women doctors counted in the Census of 1870, the large majority were still practitioners of homeopathic, eclectic, or botanic medicine. Only 137 women were enrolled in regular medical schools that year, according to the same census, which apparently ignored the irregular colleges altogether.[44]

Who were these early women physicians and what drove them to so unpromising a career? The large majority of those for whom records are available were daughters of the middle class. They were keenly sensitive to the economic changes taking place around them and the opportunities and challenges these represented. Many were deeply religious and active in reform movements to abolish slavery, intemperance, and other evils of American life. Almost all were conscious of the movement to extend women's rights, and some were involved for much of their lives in the women's movement. The great convention of women activists at Seneca Falls, New York, which framed a Declaration of Independence for women, took place while Elizabeth Blackwell was still studying at nearby Geneva College and only a year and a half before the founding of the Woman's Medical College in Philadelphia. For many reformers, the opening of medical training was a dramatic test case of their crusade to create new opportunities for women. A surprising number of the early women students, as would be true in Europe, were considerably older than their male counterparts, some were already married, and many had had experience as schoolteachers before coming to the study of medicine. Nearly all were interested in problems of women's health and hygiene and believed that women doctors could help in lifting the curtain of ignorance and superstition that surrounded the physiology of women. "I would like to be employed at something that will benefit the part of the human family that has been oppressed and suffered wrongfully," wrote a thirty-year-old woman medical student in Cincinnati, "to wit women."[45]

Even so, how was it possible for so many women to find a place to study and to engage in the active practice of medicine? What had happened to the wall of resistance that had greeted Blackwell and other pioneer women before 1850? Why was America so relatively successful in educating women doctors at a time when much of Europe still resolutely refused to allow any woman to study and practice medicine?

The explanation lies in the American political climate at mid-century and in two institutions that were largely, and at times wholly, American: the sectarian school of medicine, and the women's medical college. Whereas European medical schools, resting on the legalistic and ecclesiastical foundations of medieval Europe, were the product of deliberate state initiative, the founding of medical schools in America owed far more to private action and sponsorship. Only England of the nations of Europe, as will be described in Chapter 6, relied substantially on private enterprise and laws chartering private corporations to create a place for women in medicine. Women's reform groups in America found in the women's schools a legal means of promoting medical education for women that was largely absent in continental Europe. Any group of citizens with sufficient reason and political support could hope to gain a charter in the relaxed political environment of nineteenth-century America. In the twenty years ending in 1850 alone, the number of colleges giving medical instruction in the United States had doubled. Further, the anti-elitist sentiments of Jacksonian America had operated to remove the few restrictions on medical practice that had come out of the Revolutionary generation. Women, as well as men, could practice medicine with training that would not have passed muster in any European country.

Among the dozens of new medical schools that sprang up in the middle of the nineteenth century were special schools of homeopathy, eclectic medicine, hydropathy, and natural remedies. In Philadelphia alone, six of these unorthodox schools were founded between 1840 and 1850. The homeopathic and eclectic schools were founded on scientific principles that required a knowledge of the medical sciences which at times rivaled the requirements of the regular schools. They differed from the colleges teaching orthodox medicine, however, in their allegiance to particular theories of disease, and their avoidance of the strong drugs and bloodletting favored by the regular physicians. Although always a minority among physicians and strongly criticized by the regular profession, the sectarian doctors found favor with a broad spectrum of nineteenth-century patients. Their medical schools, often weaker and more vulnerable than the regular schools, and sometimes associated with popular health reforms, were always more open to women than those of their rivals. The National Eclectic Medical Association voted openly for a policy of coeducation in 1852. The irregular schools in Rochester, Philadelphia, New York, Cleveland, Cincinnati, and other places which admitted women all faced staggering problems of economic survival in the fierce competition among all schools for medical students. Such sectarian institutions, by admitting women to their classes, according to Regina Morantz-Sanchez, "exacerbated already bitter feelings in the regular profession."[46]

What was education like in these early irregular colleges? At some, women were separated from men as rigidly as in the women's colleges. At Penn Medical University, for example, which opened its doors in 1853, the founders stated that "a sense of propriety and delicacy cause [*sic*] us to oppose mixed or co-educational classes." Yet the training offered to women, they insisted, in contrast to that in the special colleges for women, was to be "equal to that exclusively for men." Women students would "attend no more than four lectures a day," in addition to practical exercises, in order to afford "a progressive, varied and leisurely education." Subjects taught at the school were the same as in other colleges, whether regular or irregular—anatomy, chemistry, physiology, botany, materia medica, obstetrics, surgery, and medicine. Free time "could be spent in attendance at the hospital or in study or review." Both men and women would be graduated after two full courses of lectures, which had to include a course in dissection, and two years of apprentice training "under a respectable physician."[47]

## Medical Colleges for Women

More important in the long run than the sectarian schools in accounting for the growth and acceptance of women doctors in the United States was the drive to establish regular schools of medicine for women. In all, five such schools were founded in major cities between 1850 and 1882. As early as 1848, a school for the care of women in childbirth had been started in Boston by the controversial

Samuel Gregory, who preached the need for trained women to serve the special needs of their own sex. A Yale graduate and a popular lecturer on physiology, Gregory insisted that many women stayed away from physicians out of reasons of modesty and concern for privacy. "There is no other country in the world," he wrote in 1850, "where females are so dependent upon the opposite sex for assistance on [medical] occasions."[48] He urged the revival of midwifery in America and deplored the practice of obstetrics by male physicians. "Everyone ought to wish," he said, "that the whole business of midwifery could be immediately transferred to women."[49] Reaction to his strong public crusade was mixed. While the religious press praised his campaign against "man-midwives," other papers derided his appeals. To the *Boston Herald,* for example, he was "a man of no force or originality of thought, whatever: a mere pilferer of small wares; a poor plagiarist [who] speaks in a slovenly, monotonous and halting manner, and cannot pronounce even the commonest English words correctly."[50]

Gregory's Boston school, launched as a medical college for women, was in reality confined largely to the teaching of hygiene, physiology, obstetrics, and the diseases of women. Its initial charter, granted in 1850, described its purposes as educating "Midwives, Nurses, and Female Physicians."[51] Clearly, a number of the supporters of Gregory's venture expected that the school would soon educate women doctors. At the organizational meeting in 1848, Gregory had unequivocally told the thirty men assembled that "the time has arrived to provide for the education of Female Physicians, especially for those departments that pertain to their own sex." He had searched and found, he said, "twelve intelligent and enterprising women" to begin classes and two physicians, Enoch C. Rolfe and William M. Cornell, to teach them.[52] Two years later, the group organized by Gregory to provide financial support (the Female Medical Education Society) had grown to five hundred members, including such well-known Bostonians as Horace Mann, Charles Francis Adams, and George Emerson. But all was not well at the college. The moody and zealous Gregory was frequently at odds with his supporters, including a number of powerful women, and eventually he alienated his faculty as well. Finances were frequently chaotic and enrollment in the school failed to grow. Gradually, the early hopes for the college began to fade.

The first graduates of the New England Female Medical College, as it was called, were prepared almost exclusively for the practice of midwifery. A full medical course was not even attempted until 1852, following efforts to unite the college with the medical school for women in Philadelphia the year before.[53] The first medical degrees given to women in Boston were awarded in 1854, and a small number of women continued to graduate as physicians for the next twenty years. In 1874, after Gregory's death and inconclusive efforts to unite the college with Harvard, it was merged with the homeopathic medical school of Boston University. By that time, a total of 282 women had attended the school, of whom 98 had gotten medical degrees.[54] Although clearly weaker than the other women's schools, the Boston venture nevertheless gave a sorely needed chance at medical training to a number of New England women. Among the better-known graduates were Mary Harris Thompson, the soon-to-be founder of the leading women's medical college in the Midwest, and Rebecca Lee, the first black woman to earn a medical degree in North America.

The college in Philadelphia was a far stronger venture. It grew out of Quaker benevolence and the women's reform movement in the city. Some of the early faculty members had already taken women students as apprentices. It was Philadelphia physicians, moreover, who had encouraged Elizabeth Blackwell in her search for a medical college. The Woman's Medical College of Pennsylvania (at first called the Female Medical College of Pennsylvania) opened in the fall of 1850 with a capable board of trustees, seven male faculty members, and forty students. "Our object," said the trustees in a public statement, "is not merely to qualify females as Practitioners of Medicine, but to teach 'woman to know herself,' to understand her organism, and . . . to throw open to them those avenues of Science, from which they have been so long excluded."[55] Unlike the situation at the school in Boston, it was made clear from the beginning that a full-fledged medical school for women comparable to those for men was being attempted. Although the qualifications for entrance were scanty and clinical opportunities nonexistent, the faculty and board made clear their commitment to the recommendations on medical education laid down by the recently formed American Medical Association.

The whole burden of winning goodwill for the College fell on the faculty and the active board of trustees, especially its chairman, William J. Mullin, and its secretary, Dr. Joseph Longshore.[56] It was these two, according to Longshore's brother, who "almost alone" raised the monies to start the classes.[57] Mullin, a popular jeweler, was an irrepressible enthusiast and generous benefactor of women's education who himself lacked an extensive formal education. The first graduating class, it was said, petitioned the board to ask that someone other than Mullin confer the diplomas "since he was an uneducated man."[58] If such a request was indeed made, the board understandably demurred. They were concerned with far more serious problems. Members of the faculty were teaching without pay and were increasingly concerned about using their own funds to buy supplies and to keep the enterprise going.[59] Their colleagues in the city were largely antagonistic to the College. "No reputable Doctor of any note," wrote Longshore, "would touch the work."[60] Teachers and students from other colleges also made their hostility to the women's school evident. On the day of the first graduation, five hundred male medical students and their friends crowded the ceremonial hall and threatened to disrupt the exercises. The mayor of the city, in response, was forced to assign fifty policemen to cordon off the hall and maintain peace.[61]

Among the eight women earning degrees that evening in December 1851 were Ann Preston, aged thirty-eight, destined to play a crucial role in the school's history as professor and later dean, and Hannah E. Longshore, aged thirty-two, who would teach anatomy in both Boston and Philadelphia. Longshore would be the first woman to put up her sign as a physician in Philadelphia. Seldom, however, did she hear a call for her services. "The novelty of a woman doctor," wrote her husband, "attracted the curious sometimes to her office to see what a woman doctor was, and calling under the pretense of injury for a nurse or some other improvised errand."[62] The gentle and diminutive Preston, on the other hand, never attempted to practice but joined the college as a professor of physiology in 1853. She would lead the effort to start a women's hospital in Philadelphia in 1861 so that women students, barred from other hospitals, would have a chance at clinical training. Her philosophy of life and Quaker outlook made her a quiet but persistent champion of women's right to study and practice medicine. She believed strongly that women were unalterably different from men—gentler, more sensitive, more loving—and that they should occupy a special place in the healing arts.[63] This view of woman's special place in medicine was indelibly stamped on many generations of graduates of the Philadelphia school. By the time of Preston's death in 1872, the College had survived the worst of its birthing ordeal and had graduated 138 women physicians.[64]

In the three decades after the establishment of the women's schools in Boston and Philadelphia, regular schools were also launched in New York (1865), Chicago (1870), and Baltimore (1882). The school in Baltimore came on the scene after a number of western state universities had already made the decision to admit women, but the New York and Chicago schools still benefited from the paucity of educational opportunities for women doctors.[65] The school in New York was the most ambitious of the special schools for women. From the beginning of her career in that city, Elizabeth Blackwell had struggled to gain clinical experience for herself and other women physicians. In 1857, with the help of her sister Emily and the young Marie Zakrzewska, she had started an infirmary of twenty-four beds. Recent graduates of the medical schools in Philadelphia and Boston made their way to the infirmary to gain some experience in bedside care. "The practical gain to these young women," wrote Zakrzewska later, "was so great that they were more than willing to bear great physical discomfort, as well as the ridicule which they encountered when they attempted to demand the recognition and the respect due to their calling."[66] Dissatisfied with the medical training of most of the women who came to work in the infirmary, Blackwell began efforts to create a school of high standards in New York. "We were extremely reluctant to open another college," said Emily later: "It was already easy enough for women to obtain a degree."[67] In 1865, a charter was obtained for a college that would provide a graded curriculum (then rare), sessions of six to eight months in length, obligatory clinical experience, a course in hygiene or preventive medicine, an outside board of examiners, and a three-year course of study.

In the mid-1860s scarcely any medical school in America offered more than two brief terms of four to five months each. Although some of these features could not be put immediately in place, the Woman's College of the New York Infirmary was abreast of most of its contemporaries among male medical schools. When the College did move to make three years of study obligatory in 1874, "we nearly ended the college . . . the next year our class fell to less than one half."[68] Because of the role played by the prominent Blackwells and later by Mary Putnam (Jacobi), the New York school was probably the most closely watched of all the women's medical schools. In its first decade of experience (the school opened its doors in 1868), it graduated fifty-three women physicians.[69]

Five years after Elizabeth Blackwell won a charter for her school in New York, one of her interns, the energetic Mary Harris Thompson, herself a graduate of Gregory's school in Boston, opened a women's medical college in Chicago. Thompson had been in Chicago only seven years, during which time she had succeeded in getting a second degree from the Chicago Medical College, opening a medical and surgical practice, and launching a hospital for women and children. Two other women who had enrolled with her at the Chicago Medical College had suddenly been asked to leave without finishing their studies. A sympathetic faculty member, William H. Byford, suggested the idea of a women's college in connection with the women's and children's hospital.[70] The reaction of the profession, however, was no more tolerant than it had been in the Eastern cities. Among medical men, said Dr. Byford, "it was almost a disgrace to be seen walking on the street with a woman doctor to say nothing of the enormity of showing her a kindness."[71] The medical journals were uniformly hostile, usually referring to Dr. Thompson as "Miss Doctoress Thompson," although one, perhaps grudgingly, admitted that "We do not advise women to study or practice medicine as a profession; but, to such as are determined to do so, without our advice, we say, they will find the Woman's Hospital Medical College, of Chicago, worthy of their patronage."[72] As the only regular women's medical college west of the Appalachians, the Chicago school attracted scores of would-be doctors, including such well-known figures as Sarah Hackett Stevenson, Marie Mergler, Eliza Root, Mary Bates, and Helga Rudd. It survived the loss, in the Great Fire of 1871, of the Hospital, the College, and the offices and books of three-fourths of its faculty. By the time it merged with Northwestern University two decades later, it had graduated 350 women physicians.[73]

The experiment of educating women doctors in separate schools drew both support and criticism from the medical profession. In every city, a small band of male physicians gave critical help to the women's cause by teaching in the women's schools, raising money, or speaking in their behalf. These were men like Byford in Chicago, Henry Bowditch and Samuel Cabot in Boston, and Henry Hartshorne and Alfred Stillé in Philadelphia, who, in the words of Marie Zakrzewska, "stood head and shoulders above their colleagues [and] who could afford to make enemies in and out of professional circles."[74] Others tolerated the women's colleges as a practical solution to the dilemma of giving women a chance at medical training while preserving the male character of the established schools. Still others opposed outright any effort to train women in medicine and refused to consult with them, admit them to hospitals, or allow them to join medical societies. The powerful Philadelphia County Medical Society, for example, passed a resolution forbidding members to hold professorships in the Woman's College and barring them from consulting with women practitioners.[75] The editor of the *Boston Medical and Surgical Journal* reflected perfectly the uncertain mood of the profession when he wrote in 1853:

> Female physicians seem to be on the increase among us, and establishing circles of good practice, in spite of the jeers, innuendoes and ridicule of us lords of creation . . . It is not a matter to be laughed down, as readily as was at first anticipated. The serious inroads made by female physicians in obstetrical business, one of the essential branches of income to a majority of well-established practitioners, makes it natural enough to inquire what course it is best to pursue? All the female medical colleges have charters from the same sources from which our own emanate, and the law is no respecter of persons, whether dressed in tights or bloomers, in affairs purely scientific and intellectual.[76]

Even in Europe, the pioneer American schools attracted the attention of women who were struggling for a chance at medical education. News of the college in Philadelphia, for example, reached Marie Zakrzewska in Berlin at a time when she despaired of her future and influenced her decision to emigrate to America.[77] In England, the young Elizabeth Garrett was planning in 1862 to come to America for a medical degree after finishing the work for an apothecary's license in her homeland.[78] The reformer Sophia Jex-Blake did come to the United States, to Boston, where she was introduced to the world of medicine and feminism. Any visitor to the women's hospital in Boston, she wrote home, must be "convinced of the enormous advantage of women doctors."[79] From far-off Russia came a representative of the imperial government in 1860 to inspect the

New York Infirmary and report on the medical education of women in America. The government of Alexander II was itself facing the question of how to respond to the growing number of women from middle- and upper-class families who now sought admission to medicine.[80]

All of the women's colleges had to struggle to stay alive in the face of professional scorn and harrowing financial troubles. Their buildings were old and needed constant repair; they often lacked equipment to demonstrate the lectures; they were usually wanting in clinical opportunities; and they were dependent, especially at first, on the few male faculty members who were willing to help them. The dean of the Philadelphia school later recalled that there had been no money for compensating the faculty, no medical journal that would take its advertisements, no hospital where its students were safe from insult. Men who accepted faculty appointments were themselves ostracized by many of their colleagues.[81] Of the women's school in Boston, Harriot Hunt said: "I regret to say that its standard has never been such, as to induce the highest minds to *graduate* there."[82] Marie Zakrzewska, who taught there briefly after leaving New York, deplored the low standards and finally refused to agree to the award of the M.D. degree to several women who had completed the course.[83] Mary Putnam, the harshest critic of the women's schools, described the Boston college as "ludicrously inadequate" and Philadelphia as "scarcely an improvement." Of Philadelphia, where she had herself studied, she wrote: "The instruction consisted of rambling lectures, given by gentlemen of good intentions but imperfect fitness, to women whose previous education left them utterly unprepared to enter a learned profession, and many of them were really, and in the ordinary sense, illiterate." Students at the school, she continued, went for the first twelve years of its existence with almost no chance to see sick people, which, in light of her experience in Paris, "would have been considered outrageous in any country but the United States."[84] Elizabeth Blackwell summarized the situation confronting medical women in the mid-1860s as she prepared to open her own school in New York.[85]

> We will commence the subject by one single statement—there is not in the whole extent of our country, a single medical school where women can obtain a good medical education. I trust that no one will construe this statement as an attack upon the schools already organized. We have watched their growth with deep interest; we have been

solicited to take part in most of them, and would gladly have done so, could we have conscientiously approved of them.

Yet the shortcomings of the women's schools, and of the sectarian schools, should not be overemphasized. The typical American medical school of the antebellum years, whether for men or women, whether orthodox or irregular, was woefully deficient by European standards. Many were run by ill-trained physicians who considered the education of doctors a business, and a profitable one at that. "The medical colleges of this country," the United States commissioner of education quoted a Boston physician as saying, "are mostly joint-stock corporations, who furnish as little medical education as they can sell at the highest price they can obtain."[86] Both men's and women's schools of all kinds required little in the way of preliminary education; the normal course of study was two terms of four months each; the second term was largely a repetition of the lectures given in the first; clinical experience was haphazard and far beneath European standards; and graduates were examined by no outside body. Schools outrivaled one another by cutting fees, shortening the curriculum, and establishing easy requirements for degrees. Professors often fought furiously over the division of student fees. At the Rush Medical College in Chicago, for example, a disgruntled professor resigned in 1849, saying, "It is a small potato business of which I am most heartily tired . . . The money is not divided and will not be . . . They say they pay debts . . . with the matriculation and graduation fees—but the debts are usually going to themselves."[87] No women's medical college, so far as can be determined, was charged with fiscal greed or improper use of funds. Most of the women's schools, on the contrary, sought to stretch their meager resources as far as possible to serve educational ends. The schools in New York, Philadelphia, and Chicago moved farther than most of their contemporaries in trying to extend and grade the curriculum, as well as in meeting other standards proposed by the American Medical Association.

## Segregation and Its Effects

The leading women in American medicine continued to argue for coeducation, while simultaneously trying to strengthen the women's colleges and urging their students, where possible, to go abroad. "It is almost impossible for a lady to get a *good* medical education without going to Europe," said Elizabeth Blackwell in 1863 after American women's medical schools had been in operation for a dozen years.[88] By this time, many European clinics and hospitals allowed graduate women doctors to spend brief periods in advanced study while continuing to bar women from regular medical schools. "This troublesome and expensive method," said Blackwell, "is still the only way in which a woman can obtain anything that deserves to be called a medical education."[89]

None of the pioneer women doctors believed that the women's schools were an adequate substitute for attendance at the best medical schools of America and Europe. Zakrzewska, Putnam, Thompson, and the Blackwells had all been educated, in whole or in part, in coeducational schools and never wavered in their determination to gain admission for other women. The elder Blackwell started the women's college in New York, she said, "with hesitation, for our own feeling was adverse to the formation of an entirely separate school for women."[90] Zakrzewska repeatedly decried the senselessness of separate schools. In seeking entrance to the men's colleges, she wrote, women were only seeking the best, "and it is the Best in their chosen profession that medical women have always been seeking."[91] The English pioneer Jex-Blake, despite her clinical experience at the women-controlled New England Hospital for Women and Children, eventually, after Harvard and Edinburgh had rejected her, sought her medical degree in an established university in Switzerland.[92] Other European women, such as Franziska Tiburtius of Berlin, stoutly resisted the idea of separate women's colleges on the grounds that they forced women into a permanent second-class status in medicine.[93] Many of those who completed a degree in a women's college, such as Mary Putnam, Mary Thompson, and Amanda Sanford, when given the chance, took further training and were awarded a second degree in a coeducational school.

The forced segregation of women into separate schools and hospitals left a residue of bitter pride in several generations of medical women. Unable to study in the stronger medical colleges or to intern in the larger hospitals, many women exaggerated the benefits of separate institutions and drew closer together in protection against a hostile world. At the same time, they sought to embrace the profes-

sional standards of the larger profession. For the early interns at the
New England Hospital for Women and Children, writes Virginia
Drachman, separatism "shaped almost every aspect of their professional lives," even after they had completed their training. Their
choices were after all limited: either stay at the Hospital or work in
another all-women's institution.[94] A network of close relationships
was thus forged among these women at the New England Hospital
and elsewhere. A women's medical society was organized in Boston
among the doctors at the New England Hospital.[95] Zakrzewska was
extremely close to the interns she trained in Boston and was in
frequent contact with other women doctors at home and abroad.
Blackwell, too, gave constant personal advice to dozens of medical
women on both sides of the Atlantic. Of her first meeting with Blackwell, Zakrzewska later said that "from this [day] I date my new life
in America."[96]

The ties between British and American women doctors were likewise close, and all the pioneers—Blackwell, Zakrzewska, Preston,
Putnam, Dimock, Garrett, Jex-Blake, Elizabeth Morgan—knew and
supported one another. Elizabeth Garrett had first met Blackwell in
London in 1858, for example, and had been inspired by her lectures
on "Medicine as a Profession for Ladies."[97] A decade later, Jex-Blake,
then battling the authorities at the University of Edinburgh for admission, tried to bring Mary Putnam from Paris to the Scottish city
to teach the young women who had been denied the right to study.[98]
Dimock, too, was known to the British pioneers, and her tragic death,
by shipwreck, in 1875 brought wide notice in Great Britain. Garrett
said of her: "I never knew anyone of her age, whose character
attracted me more."[99] Circumstances had of necessity forged a common alliance among women doctors on both sides of the Atlantic
against the conditions of study and practice that confronted them.

The American women who studied abroad were especially conscious of the weakness of their medical education at home. Thousands of American male physicians, beginning in the 1860s, went
to Germany and other centers in order to perfect their knowledge
of a clinical specialty or, in some cases, to learn fundamental sciences
in the laboratory. But American women went for a different reason.
They hoped to gain by foreign study the general experience in a large
hospital or clinic that was denied them at home. Only the women's

hospitals launched by Zakrzewska in Boston, by Preston in Phila-delphia, by the Blackwells in New York, and by Thompson in Chicago were freely open to women interns and individual students. But all of them offered only limited opportunities for seeing a wide range of diseases or learning the latest techniques and procedures in sci-entific medicine.

Nearly all of the pioneer women doctors in the quarter-century after 1850 went abroad for a period of clinical study. Esther Lovejoy, in her groundbreaking study *Women Doctors of the World*, writes that going abroad was the only way that the graduates of women's and sectarian colleges could "eke out their meager educational oppor-tunities."[100] The influential Blackwells, for example, both spent two years abroad after their graduation working in the Maternité hospital in Paris and in the clinics of leading physicians James Paget, James Simpson, and others.[101] The early Cleveland graduate Nancy Clark went to Paris with her physician-brother in 1854 after getting her medical degree.[102] From the Woman's Medical College of Pennsyl-vania, Emmeline Cleveland was sent by a group of Quaker women to the Maternité in 1860 to fit herself to teach obstetrics. She was followed from Philadelphia by Anna Broomall and Frances Emily White.[103]

In Boston, most of the early staff at the New England Hospital spent at least a year abroad, including Lucy Sewall, Helen Morton, Emma Call, Augusta and Emily Pope, Susan Dimock, Annette Buckel, and Mary Almira Smith.[104] Morton indeed spent four years at the Maternité, the last two as an instructor.[105] Seven of the early graduates of the women's medical college in New York went to Europe in the late 1860s and early 1870s to continue their educa-tion.[106] Similarly, in Chicago, Marie Mergler went to Zurich after graduating from the Woman's Hospital Medical College, while Eliza Root studied in Vienna to get more experience in obstetrics after her graduation.[107] Of the sixty-eight prominent nineteenth- and early-twentieth-century women physicians listed in the *Dictionary of Amer-ican Medical Biography*, thirty-two, or nearly half, spent some time in postgraduate study abroad.[108] In all, according to an earlier esti-mate by the author, between six and eight hundred American women studied abroad, chiefly in postgraduate clinics and hospitals, between 1870 and 1914.[109]

The American Achievement

Twenty years after Blackwell's entrance into the Geneva Medical College in 1847 it appeared that the United States had moved far to the forefront in the medical education of women. As yet no modern European university had graduated a single woman in medicine. The sectarian and women's colleges of medicine in America had already produced, by contrast, several hundred women doctors. Of the 544 women counted in one study, including some who held no degree, only eleven were graduates of regular coeducational medical schools before 1871.[110] The very success of the growing number of women graduates, however educated, kept the pressure constant on the regular profession. The women competed with male physicians for patients; they committed few of the predicted medical blunders; they won friends who were prominent in public life; they fought for admission to medical societies; they petitioned constantly for hospital privileges; and they continually demanded of educational authorities and male faculty members why they would not allow women to matriculate. Harvard Medical School, which had repeatedly denied admission to women, now found itself increasingly split on the question of coeducation. Public universities, especially in the western states, began seriously to consider the possibility of admitting women to medical study.

By 1870, the combined effect of the women's and sectarian colleges had opened a sizable breach in the wall of opposition to women. "The path had been broken," wrote Zakrzewska, "and the profession had been obliged to yield, and to acknowledge the capacity of women as physicians."[111] By this time, teaching in the women's schools had begun to improve, enrollment was rising, and a scattering of clinical opportunities, especially in the women's hospitals and clinics, existed in a number of cities. Although women still accounted for fewer than one percent of all physicians in the United States, the woman doctor was now less frequently seen as a lonely exception to her gender's unfitness for medicine. Among a number of male physicians, though clearly not yet a majority, the feeling was growing that women should have a chance at medical training, if only in segregated schools. The opening of the state university of Michigan to women medical students in 1870 was everywhere seen as an important milestone on the road to full equality. Meanwhile, in Europe, the example of the American pioneer doctors was being used in a number of countries in the fight to lower barriers to women.

But change was slow and halting. The schools that had educated Zakrzewska and the Blackwells were now closed to women. Harvard refused women once more, in 1867, as it would do repeatedly until 1945. Other leading medical schools followed suit. Resistance was strongest in the conservative East, where the most successful of the established schools were to be found. Where women were admitted to public universities, as in Michigan, they reported personal slights or protested the indignity of separate classes and laboratories to screen them from knowledge thought unfit for women.[112] Hospital appointments for women as interns were still almost impossible to obtain outside the few women's hospitals. Hostile reactions to women in clinics or medical classes were reported at the end of the 1860s and the beginning of the 1870s in Philadelphia, Ann Arbor, and across the Atlantic in Edinburgh. And the old argument of exceptionalism was far from dead. At the annual meeting of the American Medical Association in San Francisco in 1871, Dr. Horatio Storer said:

> We will grant that some exceptional women are as interested in our science as ourselves— . . . but, beyond this there is a point that is fundamental to the whole matter . . . and that is, this inherent quality in their sex, that uncertain equilibrium, that varying . . . according to the time of the month in each woman that unfits her for taking those responsibilities of judgment which are to control the question often of life and death.[113]

For all the flaws in the American record, however, the history of the medical education of women before 1870 is largely an American story. The medical schools and examining bodies of Great Britain were still resolutely closed to women, as were the schools of Germany, Austria, and most of Europe. Only one European woman, Elizabeth Garrett, who had secured an apothecary's license before that loophole was closed in Britain, was actually practicing medicine with official approval at the end of the 1860s. Europeans looked to the new women doctors of the United States with mixed feelings. A number of women in Europe found hope and encouragement in their achievement, but others believed that the special schools for women were a mistake. Women's schools in America, wrote a con-

tributor to *Macmillan's Magazine* in 1868, had been created "in per-
ilous haste." The "meagre curriculum, and the low standard of
examination—a standard so low indeed that it is said to be difficult
for a student *not* to get the M.D. at some of the female schools—
sufficiently explain the inferior professional position taken by most
of their graduates." The American system of medical education, said
the writer, "has produced much that is bad in the education of men;
but it has been even more injurious to women."[114]

The medical professors and physicians of Europe generally deplored the relaxed standards in America that had made possible the
creation of sectarian and women's schools. "Most of these women
doctors in America," said Professor Wilhelm von Zehender of Rostock, after corresponding with physicians in America and Europe,
"do not stand in very high regard." The state in America, he wrote,
took "no responsibility for the education and licensing of its physicians," which explained "the large number of miserable medical
schools and so-called colleges" that gave diplomas to both sexes after
a short period of lectures. A few schools, such as Harvard, tried for
a higher standard, "but at this university women are absolutely
prohibited."[115]

By 1870, several European countries had taken the first steps to
allow women to study medicine on the same basis as men. The
presence of Mary Putnam in Paris and Susan Dimock in Zurich
signaled a historic shift toward greater equality for women in medicine. The two Americans were members of the vanguard of a great
migration of medical women that affected thousands of women over
the next half-century. It was the largest migration of professional
women in history. From all over Europe, especially Russia, from
Britain and Australia, from Canada and the United States, and places
beyond, a steady stream of women seeking a first-rate medical education began to pour into Switzerland and France. The attention
that had for so long been focused on the United States in women's
medical education now began to shift across the Atlantic, especially
to the universities in Zurich and Paris.

# 2 Zurich and Paris

The names of the women who pioneered in medical study at Zurich —Suslova, Bokova, Morgan, Dimock, Atkins, Walker, and Vögtlin— are little known today. Few monuments have been raised in their memory. They are barely mentioned in the standard histories of women's early education in medicine. Compared to an Elizabeth Blackwell or a Marie Zakrzewska or a Sophia Jex-Blake, they would seem to have played only a passing role in the drama of women's battle to study medicine.

And yet these seven women, coming from four different countries, made possible the most important victory won by medical women in the nineteenth century. Their success at the University of Zurich opened the doors to the full acceptance of women as fellow students with men in a university environment. Unlike the American medical schools at Geneva and Cleveland, which quickly banned women after admitting a few, the school at Zurich remained open to women and was joined by other Swiss universities in welcoming hundreds, and then thousands, of female medical students from all over Europe and North America. Further, the Swiss schools were genuine universities, requiring five years of university-level study to graduate in medicine, in contrast to the scant eight months of practical instruction that was then the standard in American medical schools. It was in Zurich that medical coeducation was realized for the first time. Along with Paris, which followed hard on the heels of Zurich in allowing women to study medicine, the Swiss universities led the world for half a century in their openness to women.

## Rendezvous in Zurich

The crucial period came in the years after 1864. In that year, a Russian woman, Maria Kniazhnina, sought permission to attend lectures in anatomy and microscopy at the University of Zurich. The request came to a university and a city in the grip of profound social change. Both were affected by the lively democratic spirit in the canton, by the growing importance of its commercial outreach, and by the presence of an increasing number of political refugees and radical emigrés in the city. These were years, writes Gordon Craig, "in which the liberal belief in progress through freedom was still unscarred by the disappointments of a later time, years in which anything and everything seemed possible, and in which Zurich under liberal leaders seemed to have cast off the constraints of its provincial past and to be developing, for the first time, a truly intellectual character."[1] A liberal humanitarianism informed the efforts of Zurich leaders to advance the cause of educational and social reform. "Men and women," wrote the historian Theodor Mommsen of his years in Zurich, "lust after *Bildung* here as the mice do after the grease pot."[2] Among those who lusted after education in the city on the Limmat were the talented daughters of the commercial hierarchy, who from time to time were allowed to audit lectures in the new university founded in 1833. Women were also frequent visitors at the evening lectures in the university that drew a significant number of the leaders of Zurich society.[3] It was thus not without precedent that the university readily agreed to Kniazhnina's informal attendance at the anatomical and microscopical classes.[4]

Kniazhnina arrived in a city of about thirty-five thousand people that was alive with commercial bustle and political ferment. Its liberal government had modernized the cantonal capital, torn down the ancient walls that had confined the city's growth, and rebuilt the city's streets and bridges. Zurich was now the economic center of the nation with specialized facilities for international banking and credit. It stood at the fulcrum of a transportation network of railroads and steamships. Its industries were at the forefront of the entire Alpine region. In political and intellectual life, its citizens were subject to the swirling tides of reform that had emanated from France and the revolutions of 1830 and 1848. The city swarmed with political dissidents and refugees from the great powers that surrounded it.[5]

The university benefited both from the liberal government of the canton and from the stream of German refugees escaping the repressions that followed the uprisings of 1848. Its medical faculty included from the beginning a large number of German professors who had fled from the restrictive atmosphere of the German universities. The distinguished internist Johannes Schönlein had come to the university in 1833 following his suspension at Würzburg.[6] The anatomist Jakob Henle had for political reasons faced delay in getting a university appointment in Germany and had joined the Zurich faculty in 1840.[7] The pathologist Karl Ewald Hasse, who stayed in Zurich until 1852, called the city "a peaceful island in a stormy ocean."[8]

From many places came young scientists destined to play a commanding role in the changes overtaking medical science. The reputation of the university grew as it provided shelter to those awaiting major appointments in Germany. The young surgeon Theodor Billroth, who was teaching in Zurich when Kniazhnina arrived, called it "an academic waiting station first class."[9] By the 1860s, Zurich, like Bern and Basel, was an important part of the German university world. Its hospital and gynecological clinics were led by such well-known Germans as Billroth, Wilhelm Griesinger, and Adolf Gusserow.

## Nadezhda Suslova: The Russian Pioneer

The spring after Kniazhnina's arrival, a second Russian woman, the twenty-one-year-old Nadezhda Suslova, also from St. Petersburg, was allowed to attend lectures at the university. She had already learned a good deal of medicine in her native land and was now determined to finish her studies. Both she and Kniazhnina had been swept up in the wave of reforms following the Russian defeat in the Crimea and the liberation of its serfs, when for a time Russia led the continent in job and schooling opportunities for women. Education had become the passion of the Russian "women of the sixties," indispensable to their fight for economic independence and equality with men. Women had begun to attend university lectures in Russia in 1859 and by the early 1860s more than sixty women were attending courses at the St. Petersburg Medical-Surgical Academy. But a burst of student radicalism that touched a number of the women students led to their abrupt expulsion from the universities. Among those expelled was Nadezhda Suslova, destined to play a central role in the unfolding drama at Zurich.[10]

Suslova found the atmosphere in Switzerland far freer than that in her homeland. She had been born the daughter of a serf, who subsequently freed himself from indenture, in a small town near Nizhnii Novgorod. Her mother, who was unusually well educated for her class, began teaching her early in life. Her ambitious father, with the help of his employer, Count Shermetev, saw to it that Nadezhda and her sister (later a good friend of Dostoevsky) got a good basic education. In the 1860s the Suslovas moved to St. Petersburg, where Nadezhda was caught up in the movement for the emancipation of women in the capital city. She attended the lectures of some of the best-known professors at the University of St. Petersburg. She was active in a section of the revolutionary "Land and Freedom" movement. With the help of the sympathetic physiologist Ivan Sechenov, she won permission to study as an auditor at the Medical-Surgical Academy. But her studies in anatomy and physiology at the Academy were cut off by the government's ban on further study by women, and she then made the decision to go to Zurich.[11]

She knew that a number of Russians were already studying in the Swiss city. Doubtless she knew, too, that Kniazhnina had been admitted to medical lectures the preceding winter. It was common knowledge that Zurich, like most European universities, demanded little of its foreign students in the way of preparatory education. Foreigners were allowed to enter with little formal preparation but were then expected to meet the same rigorous examination standards as native students. Nowhere else in the world, in any case, was it possible for a woman to take her place in medical lectures in a recognized university.

But would Zurich allow her to take a medical degree? For a time both Kniazhnina and Suslova continued as auditors in the university, while the Academic Senate was divided on the question of whether women could be fully matriculated. Kniazhnina left the university for reasons that are not clear, but Suslova took the bold step in 1867 of requesting permission to take the examinations for a medical degree. The Zurich faculty and cantonal government were now forced to face squarely the issue of women at the university. The zeal and perseverance of the shy Russian woman had made a strong impression on the professors and students. She had fulfilled all the conditions for the examinations except formal matriculation. The educational authorities of the canton turned the issue back to the faculty. In their discussions it became clear that the largely German faculty, especially the new internist Anton Biermer, who had replaced Griesinger, and the politically liberal physiologist Adolf Fick, were determined to give the Russian woman a chance. They advised the university rector to take the position that it was senseless to debate the issue of Suslova's right to be examined when she was not yet formally enrolled in the University. He followed their advice, admitted her retroactively to 1865, and thus made her eligible to take the required examinations, an eligibility that no one now contested.[12]

It was a crucial decision. Suslova's request had fallen on ground made fertile by three decades of liberal reform in Zurich. Nowhere in Europe or America could so liberally minded and sympathetic a medical faculty have been assembled to hear the case for women's education. In addition to Biermer and Fick, the faculty in 1867 included Billroth and his assistant and successor Edmund Rose, the fatherly Hermann von Meyer, professor of anatomy, the gynecologist Gusserow, the pathologist Carl Eberth, the liberal ophthalmologist Friedrich Horner, and the histologist and 1848 refugee Heinrich Frey.[13] So far as the faculty records indicate, no one opposed vocally the move to admit a woman to full matriculation in the university. In the Academic Senate, the medical faculty had the support of other professors, especially the political economist Victor Böhmert, who became a lifelong champion of women's rights in education and the chronicler of Zurich's pioneering role in admitting women.[14]

But it was Suslova herself whose quiet abilities triggered a sympathetic response in the faculty. She lived unobtrusively in Zurich and worked very hard. Some lectures started as early as six A.M. and the day did not end until the early evening. She had few friends outside the Russian emigré community. Like many in her generation of Russian women, she was an ardent feminist and a follower of the nihilistic doctrines sweeping her homeland, and believed strongly in serving the common people of Russia. Switzerland had been particularly recommended to her because it was the freest country in

Europe and far removed from the Russian police. A countrywoman recalled her surprise in meeting her: "I expected an energetic, confident personality. The opposite was the case. She had a quiet, serious temperament with deep feelings and a thoughtful, melancholy look from somewhat deep-set brown eyes."[15] A fellow student, the Swiss psychiatrist August Forel, described her as "quite shy."[16] The pathologist Rindfleisch, who taught her at Zurich, said that "she was in her manner so modest that no one had the slightest reason to complain but at the same time diligent, very skillful in making microscopic preparations; her questions and answers showed a complete understanding of what was going on. I was very satisfied with this pupil."[17]

What must it have been like for this pioneer woman? She was now the only officially enrolled woman in the entire university; her native land lay a thousand miles to the east; the German language was difficult for her and she had trouble expressing herself; the study was arduous and the system different from what she had known in St. Petersburg; her future on returning to Russia was uncertain; and for a time she was the only woman in the world studying for a medical degree under the same conditions as men. In a letter home, she wrote of her feelings of isolation and her constant immersion in books.[18] She did become friendly with an idealistic Swiss medical student, Friedrich Erismann, and there must have been happy moments in her final year at Zurich. The meeting with Suslova was to change Erismann's life. She interested him in the painful social conditions in Russia, in the great opportunities for public health work, and filled him with the burning sense of indignation that motivated her. He became a socialist, studied public health in Germany, married Suslova in 1868 (they later divorced), and then spent much of his life in Russia as a pioneer in public hygiene, directing the first great investigations of factories and workers' lives. At one time, he held the highest position in public health in the Russian Empire.[19]

Suslova meanwhile passed the difficult qualifying examinations for the medical degree in the summer of 1867. She then went to Graz to write her thesis under the direction of her old friend Sechenov, whose reputation in physiology was growing. She returned to Zurich to defend her thesis on the physiology of the lymphatic system in December 1867. On the fourteenth day of that month, flanked by the rector of the university and the dean of the medical faculty, she slowly entered the examining room, which was filled to overflowing. Behind her marched the entire medical faculty, who took their places around the long green examining table. She was twenty-four years old, dressed in a simple black dress, shy and somewhat nervous. In her heavily accented German, she read a summary of her thesis. There followed sharp questioning from the surgeon Edmund Rose, the physiologist Ludimar Hermann, and other members of the faculty. In the words of a professor who was present, it was "no empty ceremony." Several of her interpretations were attacked but she defended her views strongly, using observations from her own research. At the conclusion, Professor Rose congratulated her on her performance and lauded the experiment in women's education. Her thesis, said Rose, proved the aptitude of women for scientific work better than any theoretical discussion of the woman question. "Soon," he said, "we are coming to the end of slavery for women, and soon we will have the practical emancipation of women in every country and with it the right to work."[20] It was the first medical degree awarded to a modern woman in a recognized university of high academic standards. "I am the first," wrote Suslova, "but not the last. After me will come thousands."[21]

Word of Suslova's success sped across Europe and America. Even before her final examination, two Englishwomen were allowed to matriculate in the fall of 1867. Both Frances Elizabeth Morgan and Louisa Atkins had lived in London; both had received a far better education than the typical Englishwoman of that era; and both realized the hopelessness of seeking a medical degree at home. Morgan had been studying medicine with private teachers and had passed the preliminary examinations for an apothecary's license before the governing council of Apothecaries Hall had moved to bar women from licensure.[22] Atkins was a young widow who had lost her husband in India and now tried to fill the painful void in her life by hard work and service to others. Unlike the cool and self-possessed Morgan, Atkins was an unusually friendly, gentle woman who knew little science and was discouraged by the difficulties of medical study.[23] She had, wrote Forel in a contemporary letter, "a much less elevated sense of herself" than her countrywoman.[24] Only by dint of extraordinary self-discipline was she able to finish her degree, including a thesis on pulmonary gangrene in children, in the normal five years.

## The Legend of Frances Elizabeth Morgan

But Morgan became a legend through her prodigies of achievement. She did as much as sixty hours of work each week at the university (including a course in Sanskrit), finished her medical work in three years, and impressed students and faculty members alike with her regal bearing and cool intelligence. After a childhood in a minister's family in Wales, she had been allowed to attend schools in Paris and Düsseldorf, then had commenced the study of medicine. When she was denied permission to take the apothecaries' examination, she left for Zurich, "hoping to breathe freer and purer air than seemed possible in England, where the medical profession was heaping its anathemas . . . on those women who chose the profession of medicine as a career."[25] Her crisp and authoritative manner both amused and irritated her fellow students. When she took her place alone in the anatomical laboratory, according to Forel, "we found this rather comical, but the seriousness, the aristocratic calm, and the royal superiority of this remarkable girl exacted such respect from all of us that none of us would have dared to make a tactless or sarcastic remark." The well-disposed anatomist Hermann von Meyer, trying to protect her modesty, suggested that certain demonstrations were "not decorous or respectable for a lady" but Morgan replied: "Herr Professor, it is much more shocking and improper to make exceptions here."[26] Within months, she was treated by her male colleagues as an equal. According to Forel, she became more and more like a man: "elle devient de plus en plus synonyme d'un étudiant du sexe masculin."[27]

Three years after Suslova, Morgan became the second woman to defend her thesis before the entire faculty. By this time other women had entered the university and interest in the medical women was running high. Morgan's reputation and the hint of disagreement with her thesis director, Anton Biermer, added to the interest. On the twelfth of March, 1870, the examination room was filled half an hour before the ceremony was scheduled to begin.[28] The faculty decided to move the examination to the Aula, the largest auditorium in the university, to accommodate colleagues and eager students. This room, too, was quickly filled with more than four hundred spectators, including fifty women who came to support their candidate. At twenty minutes after eleven o'clock the main doors opened and all eyes turned to the attractive young Englishwoman, of medium height, clad in a long black dress, who entered the auditorium accompanied by the university rector and the dean of the medical faculty. She took her seat next to the podium as Professor Rose welcomed the crowd and read her *curriculum vitae*. She then read in a low voice a summary of her thesis on progressive muscular atrophy, which had been directed by Professor Biermer.

As the discussion opened, Biermer stood up to deliver a lengthy criticism of the principal conclusions, which differed from his own published views. Those present differed on how long Biermer spoke, Forel recalling twenty-five minutes, another professor estimating only ten minutes. But all agreed it was a sharp, sometimes angry, attack and tension mounted in the auditorium. "I can still see the cool demeanor [of Morgan]," Forel later wrote, "who made notes constantly as Biermer spoke and then responded in a half-hour address until Biermer had had enough."[29] She made it clear in her English-accented remarks that she had used English and American sources not available to Biermer, and that this was the cause of the disagreement. The next questions came from the ranks of the students, as was customary, and they were answered, according to one source, with "quiet, measured, and clear responses." Biermer expressed his satisfaction with her replies and added: "You have, honored Fräulein, an important role in the solution of the great social problem that has occupied us here in Zurich. By your scholarly earnestness and zeal, you have become a worthy model for the women studying here." There followed the ceremonial awarding of the degree and a speech by Professor Rose. "My dear girl," he began, "I greet you for the first time as a colleague. I cannot refrain from expressing to you out of a full heart my appreciation for your efforts and your tact. I am glad to confirm . . . that you have given a new guarantee of the success of the social experiment being made quietly here in Zurich, an experiment that affects . . . the whole world." It had been, said Forel in an understatement, "a remarkable day."[30]

The fourth and fifth women to study medicine in Zurich arrived in the summer of 1868. Each was influenced by the previous success of women from her own country. Maria Bokova had known Suslova in St. Petersburg, where both had been active in the "Land and Freedom" movement and both had studied at the Medical-Surgical Academy before the ban against women. The other, Eliza Walker of

Edinburgh, knew of the early successes of Atkins and especially Morgan at Zurich. Walker was younger than the other pioneers, only nineteen when she began her medical studies. Less is known of her early life—only that she was born in India and was educated at the Ladies' College in Cheltenham[31]—but Forel reports that she was well liked and calls her "la très jolie Ecossaise" in a letter to his mother. She spent four years in Zurich and passed her final examination with special distinction. Her thesis on blockage of the arteries of the brain, directed by Biermer, relied on fourteen cases she had seen at the Zurich clinic as well as a thorough search of the literature. While still a student, she became the first woman assistant in the Zurich cantonal hospital, working in the women's ward.[32]

Maria Bokova, like Suslova, was well known to the Russian women of the 1860s. The daughter of a general and large landowner, she came into contact with the revolutionary movement in the early 1860s.[33] She was deeply immersed in nihilistic ideas and extraordinarily idealistic, and saw medicine as a way to serve her people. She was the model for Chernyshevsky's heroine in his influential novel *What Is to Be Done?* The oldest of the pioneers, she was twenty-nine when she enrolled at Zurich, but nevertheless showed great energy and perseverance in her studies. Some of the male students found her difficult and unfriendly—Forel said she had the same cheekiness as Morgan but none of her manners—but none doubted her ability.[34] The first Swiss woman in the medical school, Marie Vögtlin, on the other hand, wrote her mother that "Mme. B." made a deep personal impression upon her: "She is an unusually fine-looking, attractive lady with the loveliest manner that one can imagine."[35] Bokova became interested in ophthalmology and worked under Professor Friedrich Horner in studying all cases of hypopyon-keratitis at the eye clinic during the preceding ten years. Before graduating, she volunteered (along with Forel), to go to the Franco-Prussian battlefield near Belfort in 1871 with a medical expedition organized by Professor Rose. According to Rose, Bokova, who was the only woman on the expedition, "won all hearts by her steady and self-sacrificing efforts in behalf of the wounded."[36] In the fall of that year, she left Zurich to return to her native land.

The final members of the Zurich Seven were the young American Susan Dimock and the Swiss pioneer Marie Vögtlin. They arrived in Zurich in the fall of 1868 and soon became fast friends. Dimock, born in North Carolina but now living in Boston, had decided at age thirteen she wanted to be a physician like her grandfather. After her father's death, she and her mother had moved to Massachusetts to be near relatives. Like so many of the early women doctors, Dimock taught school for a while as she studied medicine from books suggested by Dr. Zakrzewska in Boston. She went to the New England Hospital to work and learn in January 1866. Both Zakrzewska and Dr. Lucy Sewall were impressed by her intellect and aptitude for medicine. After being refused admission at Harvard Medical School in 1867—as was her English fellow student at the hospital, Sophia Jex-Blake—she was encouraged by Zakrzewska and Sewall to go to Zurich in 1868.[37] Her letter of inquiry was answered by Biermer, who told her "there exists in this University no lawful impediment to the matriculation of female students and [they] enjoy equal advantages with male students."[38]

## First American: Susan Dimock

Dimock was twenty-one years old when she arrived in Zurich. Mary Putnam, who met her in Paris, urged her to spend a few days in the French capital, but Dimock refused "for the reason, which she gave me with the utmost frankness, that she had been obliged to borrow money [from Zakrzewska] in order to prosecute her studies and should not feel justified in spending a cent of it for amusement or sightseeing." She was, wrote Putnam with irony, "as fresh and girlish as if such qualities had never been pronounced by competent authorities to be incompatible with medical attainments."[39] But beneath the softness was a hardness of purpose and an almost Puritanical devotion to her work. "The American is a remarkably finished person for her age," wrote Marie Vögtlin soon after meeting her, "she looks so soft and child-like and yet there is a strong determination in her thinking and behavior."[40] Vögtlin and Dimock often studied together in the evening, Vögtlin teaching the American German, Dimock helping Vögtlin with her medical studies. Vögtlin wrote to her mother that the little band of pioneers was forming a close circle and "will stay closely together."[41] All of them realized the great stakes involved in the Zurich experiment. Here, as earlier in the United States, the first women graduates formed close and enduring friendships with one another.

Vögtlin, as the first Swiss woman, faced even greater obstacles than the others. She was forced to meet a higher admission standard than the foreigners and, unlike them, wanted to practice medicine in Switzerland itself. Critics raised the same arguments against her that were familiar in England, Russia, and America. She lacked the temperament and physical strength to practice medicine; her sex unsuited her for study alongside men; and she was abandoning home and hearth to pursue a man's vocation. "Let a few foreign women be so shameless and study," her biographer summarized the reaction, "a Swiss woman should not and must not."[42] She had been born the daughter of a minister in a conservative farm community in Argau and grown up in a family that valued books and education. At age seventeen she had been engaged to Friedrich Erismann, the same man who would later marry Nadezhda Suslova. Erismann had encouraged her intellectual and political interests, and after the breakup of their relationship Marie determined to become a physician. Her father at first reluctantly agreed but then retreated in the face of strong family and community opposition that erupted into a national outcry. Finally, however, he consented and supported his daughter in the bitter contest that followed. The university admitted her without difficulty in the fall of 1868. Her sense of responsibility for her controversial decision to study medicine brought her anguish. "I want to break new pathways," she wrote a friend, "will I succeed? The responsibility I have taken on myself is great. I feel that I stand here in the name of my entire sex and if I do poorly I can become a curse to my sex."[43]

Both Dimock and Vögtlin, like those who had come before, found the professors friendly and the students supportive. "Oh, it is so nice to get here," Dimock wrote her mother soon after her arrival, "at a word, what I have been begging for in Boston for three years."[44] The professors, she wrote her former mentor, Samuel Cabot, "are extremely kind, and take a personal interest in one's improvement . . . And the students are quiet, friendly and polite."[45] A few weeks later, she confided to her mother: "I think I shall all my life feel the advantages of having come here, where I am admitted on an equal footing with men students."[46] Soon she was making friends—Forel, Bokova, the English women, and, of course, Vögtlin. Marie Vögtlin herself was ecstatic about her reception at the university. The rector, she wrote, is "like a guardian angel to me; the professors are all extremely friendly; concerning the students all one hears [from the other women students] is how decently they treat the women."[47] Soon after her arrival she met Albert Heim, a future geology professor, whom she would marry after her graduation. And her relationship with "Miss Dimock," whom Vögtlin now called her "faithful companion," deepened as they made plans to visit Vögtlin's family and hike in the mountains over the holidays. "Miss Dimock and I," she told a friend, "are probably the best in the entire anatomy class."[48]

Dimock finished her studies and left Zurich in 1871. The parting between the two friends was painful, "like dying," said Vögtlin, "for we will probably never see each other again." The American's examination for the medical degree, the fourth after Suslova, Morgan, and Bokova, had gone well. She ably defended her thesis, done under the gynecologist Adolf Gusserow, on the different forms of puerperal fever as she had observed them in the lying-in clinic. She was highly praised by the anatomist Meyer for her energy and strong persistence. In behalf of his colleagues, he told her that it had been a special pleasure for all of them to offer the help she could not get at home. The friendly reaction of the male students, he said, had smoothed the way for their female companions.[49]

Vögtlin was the last of the little band to finish her doctorate. Unlike the others, she had had no previous training in medicine before enrolling at Zurich. After completing her course work, she took advanced study in Leipzig, where she found the German students "repulsive" in their loud and insulting behavior toward women. She then went to Dresden, where she wrote her thesis under the direction of the gynecologist Franz von Winckel, who was almost alone among German professors in supporting the aspirations of medical women. On the eleventh of July, 1874, she passed her thesis defense in the same room in Zurich where all but Morgan had preceded her.[50]

In the meantime, dozens of other women had crowded into the lecture halls and rooming houses overlooking the town of Zurich. The success of Suslova and Bokova made them heroic figures in the Russian homeland and in the other nations under Russian domination. English and American women got set to follow the example of Morgan and Dimock in seeking a first-rate university education in medicine. The first German women appeared in the early 1870s. As yet, no other nation in the world had opened its doors so fully to women medical students. The Russian women, in particular, found in Zurich an El Dorado for their hopes and ambitions. More than a hundred women, the large majority of them Russian, had taken their places in the medical school by 1873.[51]

## The Russian Crisis

The unexpected onslaught of women brought the only real crisis in the Zurich experiment. Many of the Russians were young and ill-prepared. Some of them were as young as sixteen or seventeen and had had little opportunity for academic study. The regulations at Zurich still required only a character reference from foreigners who wanted to study. Many of the newcomers were sympathetic to radical movements at home and saw medicine as the perfect outlet for serving the people. Cut off from their families in many cases, they lived cheaply in attic rooms, ate little, and seldom mixed with the towns-people of Zurich.[52] Some dressed in the characteristic costume of rebellion of the day—drab dresses, huge leather belts, short hair, round sailor hats, large blue eyeglasses—and many smoked openly on the streets.[53] In response to a query from Samuel Cabot, Susan Dimock described her own reactions to the Russian women:[54]

> Of course among 100 women a few must be found whose aims are not so high, yet very many showed a nobleness of purpose and an unselfishness of life which cannot be overlooked. Many were very rich, but ready to sacrifice in order to help the poor, their own riches and comfort and pleasure. Thus the proprietress of large tracts of country and whole villages passed the bleak Swiss winter without a flannel undergarment, saying that she would not spend her money on herself when so many poor people shivered in rags. This young girl was 16 years old, and had come to Switzerland as did most of her companions, that she might be free to work for what they call "the cause," viz. for the freedom of the people, for the social amelioration of the lower classes, better wages, better education, etc. Since these women would themselves in this matter be in no wise gainers in any tangible way, since they risked cheerfully their lives "in carrying to Russia 3 times yearly" as the Russian Government states, "incendiary letters and documents," their unselfishness cannot be doubted.

The Russian women evoked strong reactions in Zurich. A wave of protest swept over the student body at their lack of preparation, their "clannishness," and the crowding in the laboratories. Newspapers took up the attack. The sight of women and young girls walking without chaperones on Zurich streets was especially shocking. Many townspeople were incensed by their political agitation, their association with known radicals in Zurich, and the common knowledge that some were watched by Russian secret police. Others questioned the seriousness of their interest in academic matters. Still others, however, withheld judgment, expressed sympathy, or painted a more balanced picture of this first group of Russian women abroad. Franziska Tiburtius, who arrived from Germany in 1871, wrote that "despite all the craziness, martyrdom, self-importance, and lack of manners" of the Russian women, they had "honest enthusiasm, believed in their cause, and could make sacrifices for an idea." She praised their "extraordinary altruism" and eagerness to serve the less fortunate. She felt sorry, she said, that so many "intelligent, temperamental, and talented women" should be so misunderstood.[55] Another German woman, visiting in Zurich, left an affectionate portrait of a young Russian mother pushing her young child in a baby carriage up the steep route to the medical school: "Mama goes into the anatomy lab—while the child suns itself in the gardens adjoining the University."[56]

How deeply were the Russian women really involved in the radical cause? One writer has estimated the proportion of the Russian women who actively took part at ten percent. Most of them, she writes, were circumspect in their actions, stayed close to their studies, and were not sought by the police.[57] Another scholar has stated flatly that "the desire to serve society, through medical education, was the primary motivation of the majority of Russian women who had migrated to Zurich."[58] Even the revolutionist Vera Figner, who would later be sentenced to death for her role in the assassination of Alexander II, was deadly serious about her studies in medicine. "At my arrival in Zurich," she wrote, "I was possessed by one idea—to give myself entirely to the study of medicine, and I crossed the threshold of the University with a feeling of awe . . . I was nineteen years old, but I intended to renounce all pleasures, however little, in order not to lose one minute of valuable time."[59]

Among the students and townspeople of Zurich, the easy admission of foreigners to the medical school was particularly controversial. Should Zurich continue the traditional practice of welcoming foreign students from different educational systems? In the case of women, many of the Russians had not been allowed to take in their homeland the university-preparatory courses completed by men. Marie Vögtlin, along with Dimock, Bokova, Morgan, and some of the other pioneer women, tried to mediate the crisis by petitioning the Academic Senate to require women to have a preparatory education equal to that of the Swiss men. They feared that the experiment in women's education would fail "if young and immature girls without sufficient preparation and seriousness" continued to be admitted.[60] But the faculty and local government stood firm against the idea of different standards for foreign women from those for foreign men. They also resisted demands for sharp restrictions on the number of all foreign students.

The crisis was broken only when the Russian government itself published a ban against further study by women in Zurich in June 1873, arguing that the Russian radicals in the city—Bakunin and Lavrov were among them—were "luring" the young and impressionable medical women "into their net." The women had put aside scientific pursuits in favor of political agitation, the government charged; they had behaved in an undignified way; and there was concern in Russia for the next generation that would be raised by them. "The government cannot accept the idea," the decree concluded, "that two or three doctor's degrees can balance the evil which springs from the moral decay of the young generation, and therefore considers it necessary to put an end to this abnormal movement."[61] All degrees obtained by women in Zurich after 1 January 1874, according to the decree, would be invalid in Russia.

The Russian *ukase* ended the sudden torrent of female migration to the medical school at Zurich. When the fall term opened in 1873, only 18 women remained of the 104 officially enrolled the preceding semester. All but 8 of the Russian women had left Zurich in obedience to the Tsar's order.[62] They had scattered to Bern (20), Paris (11), Geneva (4), and the Russian homeland itself. About one-fourth of the Russian women eventually completed their medical degrees.[63] Most returned to Russia, either to practice medicine or midwifery or else to engage in political activity. The lives of many of them ended in tragedy. At least 22 of the former Zurich students were arrested and sentenced to prison, while others remained under close state supervision. Three died in prison, 4 committed suicide.[64] A number of them, however, were able to practice medicine and after 1878 to call themselves "doctor" following the heroic service of some in the Russo-Turkish War.

By the time the Russian crisis was resolved, the Zurich experiment was clearly a success. Never again would a serious question be raised about the admission of women in Zurich. In addition to Zurich, the medical school in Bern and the school of midwifery in Geneva were now accepting foreign women for study. Outside Switzerland, however, except for France, restrictions on the medical education of women continued in most major countries for the rest of the century. As late as 1907, neither Germany, Britain, Russia, nor the United States had opened its medical schools to women as widely as had Switzerland nearly forty years before.

The professional way in which the Swiss professors treated their women students, despite personal doubts and skepticism about co-education, set them apart from most of their colleagues in Europe and America. Many of the Swiss medical faculty regarded the education of women as an experiment, in which some of the prevailing ideas about women—their intellectual inferiority, their physical weakness, their fickleness, and their effect on male students—could be tested. The results were unexpectedly positive. Said one contemporary professor: "The presence of women, when they possess the appropriate educational background, does not disturb either the lecturers or the male students."[65] Professor Albert Heim went further in his judgment that "their presence exerts a wholesome influence on student performance and discipline that I would no longer want to do without."[66] The question of women's intellectual and physical capacity for medicine, at least so far as the Swiss were concerned, was decided by the performance of the pioneers. Of the first six women graduated at Zurich, Böhmert reports, four were evaluated as "good" and two as "very good."[67] Other Zurich professors—Forel, Rose, Meyer, Frey—spoke out in support of the medical education of women. Rose spoke for many of them when he declared: "What Zurich claims is to have been the first university to have continually opened its doors to women and thereby to have conducted the crucial experiment [*experimentum crucis*] in solving the woman question."[68]

Once convinced, the faculty and the canton never turned back in their defense of women in medicine. They examined but rejected the American alternative of separate schools for women. "Men will always regard such separate women's schools with mistrust and small regard,'' said Rose, and they will attract at best ''only mediocre faculty'' as well as students. ''Women students,'' he insisted, ''want and must have, not instructors of the second and third rank but professors of the first rank and not only in one or two but in all universities.''[69] August Forel, student and later professor at Zurich, denounced women's colleges ''as a mistaken and unnecessarily costly undertaking for Europeans.'' ''It would split forces everywhere,'' he said, ''and promote mediocrity.''[70] Other Zurich professors responded at length to criticisms from foreign colleagues and gave information to medical schools in Europe and America considering coeducation. When Theodor Bischoff launched his withering attack on women studying medicine in Zurich and America, it was the Zurich physiologist Ludimar Hermann who gave the most effective reply. Although highly skeptical himself of the spread of women's education, he defended the Zurich experiment and the women who studied there. ''Many women here,'' wrote Hermann, ''have won the high respect of teachers and fellow students by their diligence and energy.'' The lectures, he said, had not been diluted because of the presence of women. To Bischoff's argument of woman's inferiority because of her smaller brain, Hermann replied that it was known to every anatomist and physiologist that brain weight was not a measure of intellectual ability. He warned against allowing feelings alone to dictate the terms of debate about women's suitability for medicine. To advise a daughter or a sister against medicine was one thing, but for those who make laws or teach, ''the emotional standpoint does not exist.'' For his part, he urged only that the women being admitted to medical school have comparable credentials with men. ''The experiment,'' he concluded, ''has been carried out up to now with care and dignity.''[71]

## The Opening of Paris

When the Russian government stopped the flow of women to Zurich, many looked to other European schools to further their studies in medicine. A considerable number of the Russian women, as noted earlier, found a haven in Bern. Letters were sent to dozens of other universities, many in Germany, inquiring whether they would accept women for medical study. A few responded that under certain conditions it might be possible. But the Russian women who journeyed to Prague, Leipzig, Leyden, and other cities were doomed to disappointment. In Prague, the women were told that they could attend lectures but would not be allowed to graduate. A favorable decision at Leipzig seemed possible when the dean of the medical faculty recommended their admission, but the university's senate turned down his recommendation. At Leyden, the Dutch professors were sympathetic except for the professor of obstetrics, who barred them from attending his clinics and lectures.[72] One woman, Adelaide Lukanina, even made the long trip to America to work with Zakrzewska in Boston and finish her medical degree at the Woman's Medical College in Philadelphia.[73]

Outside Switzerland, only the medical school in Paris was consistently open to European women in the early 1870s. Even here, the band of Russian women found obstacles to their admission. With nearly a dozen applications from the Zurich exiles on his desk, the minister of education turned to the Russian ambassador for advice. At first the counsel from the Russian embassy was negative, but gradually the ambassador was won over to the women's cause by one of the Zurich women who had begun tutoring his children. In the end, all who applied were admitted.[74]

The Russians swelled the number of medical women in Paris to eighteen in the academic year 1873–74.[75] The first women had been admitted five years earlier when Mary Putnam, joined soon after by the Englishwoman Elizabeth Garrett, a Russian named Ekaterina Goncharova, and a Frenchwoman named Madeleine Brès, was allowed to matriculate officially in 1868. Although many faculty members were opposed, the dean of the medical faculty, Adolphe Wurtz, and the minister of education, Victor Duruy, were both sympathetic to the education of women in medicine.[76] Wurtz, who was aware of what was happening in Zurich, encouraged Madeleine Brès to finish her baccalaureate studies so that she could be admitted to the medical school, while Duruy was deeply involved in the late 1860s in plans to create a medical school for women to serve the Moslem communities in Algeria and other parts of the French Empire.[77]

The background of the first women at Paris was as varied as that of the Zurich pioneers. The first Russian woman, Goncharova, made little impression in Paris and was overshadowed at home by the pioneers who went to Zurich. All that is known about her is that she left Paris for Bern in 1870 but returned to Paris several years later to graduate in 1877. The others, however, all played a critical role in opening the medical profession to women in their homelands. Mary Putnam, as we have seen, had completed degrees in pharmacy and medicine in the United States before she arrived in Paris in 1866. She was seeking in Paris an education in medicine, according to a contemporary, "that was absolutely unattainable in the United States."[78] With the help of Duruy, she was able to surmount the opposition of the Paris faculty. After gaining full admission in 1868, she spent the next three years in hard study before passing the five required examinations and winning a coveted bronze medal for her doctoral thesis.[79] Said the *Archiv de Médecine* in its July 1871 edition:[80]

> A small event has just taken place in the Faculty of Medicine in Paris, which, although passing in a purely professional circle, is not without importance at large. A woman doctor has had her name inscribed on our registers . . . Mlle. Putnam is English by birth, French by her free choice. There is not one among us who has not been a witness to her assiduous zeal as a student. She was to be seen everywhere that there was any opportunity to learn.

While in Paris, Putnam became friends with Elizabeth Garrett. Although Putnam had been the first to matriculate, Garrett would be the first to win a degree in Paris. An extremely confident and self-possessed woman, Garrett had grown up in London and Suffolk, where her father was a successful early Victorian industrialist. She had benefited from her hard-driving father's determination to educate his daughters as well as his sons. As a young woman she was influenced by the reformer Emily Davies, who encouraged her to become a physician, arguing that "we cannot help observing many physicians and surgeons who do not appear to be superior in ability to average women."[81]

Over the objection of relatives and friends, Garrett spent six arduous months as a surgical nurse in Middlesex Hospital in London in 1860. She hoped in this way to get into the medical school run by the hospital. Although she was allowed to attend some lectures at the school and to view some demonstrations in the wards, the regular anatomy course was closed to her, so she dissected privately, in "bits and pieces," in her bedroom. In the end, however, she was rejected by the medical school because "the lecturers dislike the presence of women" and the students had organized in protest against her. In a familiar complaint, the students argued that "the presence of young females as passive spectators in the operating theatre is an outrage on our natural instincts" and would "destroy those sentiments of respect and admiration with which the opposite sex is regarded by all right minded men."[82] After being refused at other London medical schools and by St. Andrews University in Scotland, she was able through private study to pass the examinations for an apothecary's license in 1865 before that avenue to medical practice was also closed to women.

After several years of practice, Garrett determined to seek a prestigious Paris degree, providing that she would be allowed to take the examinations without becoming a full-time student. With the help of Duruy and the British ambassador, she got the necessary permission. Over the next eighteen months she passed all five of the examination hurdles and prepared to defend her thesis (on migraine) in June 1870. A last effort was made by Parisian opponents to stop the awarding of this first degree to a woman, but again they were overruled by Minister Duruy.[83] The Paris correspondent of the *Lancet* told his countrymen about her final conquest:[84]

> In great haste I write you a few lines touching the medical event of the day—to wit the reception of Miss Garrett as an M.D. of the Paris Faculty, which has just this instant taken place . . . The hall was literally crowded with students, and on Miss Garrett's crossing the courtyard to leave the school, I observed with pleasure that almost all the students gallantly bowed to their lady confrère. All the judges, on complimenting Miss Garrett, more or less expressed liberal opinions on the subject of lady doctors, and one Professor M. Broca was especially energetic and enthusiastic.

The liberal reformer Paul Broca, a surgeon and pioneer anthropologist, was one of the strongest supporters of women on the Paris faculty. He had already encouraged the career of Madeleine Brès, who, as the only French woman in the medical school, faced special barriers of the kind that had confronted Vögtlin in Zurich. Should a French woman be allowed to apply for an externship, a highly sought hospital position that involved work while still a student under supervision of members of the faculty? Would a woman be able to become an intern and serve as a house officer in one of the great hospitals of Paris? For a physician planning to carry on a practice in Paris, or to be welcome in any of its hospitals, these were important questions.

During the siege of the city in 1870–71, Brès, whose husband was serving in the national guard and who was herself responsible for three small children, asked to be assigned provisionally to one of the overworked hospitals of Paris. Broca got her a temporary position as intern at the Pitié hospital, where she remained during the Prussian onslaught. For her service during six bombardments of the hospital, she was praised by the hospital's director and a number of members of the faculty. Said Dean Wurtz of her performance: "By her ardor and hard work, by her zeal in the service of the hospital, Mme. Brès has justified the opening of our courses to students of the female sex and won the respect of all the students with whom she worked."[85] Despite this warm commendation, however, she was still denied permission, once the war had ended, to enter the competition for an externship. The official in charge told her that if it were "only she personally" who was involved, she would "probably" have been approved, but that the concern over precedent made it impossible. Full equality for women in the competition for externships and internships in France lay more than a decade in the future. In the meantime, Madeleine Brès was awarded the M.D. degree and allowed to begin practice in 1875.

The opening of Paris to medical women was not accomplished without a bitter fight. More than in Zurich, the hostility of the medical profession to women was open and public. Neither did the medical faculty rally to the women's cause as had happened in Zurich. "Paris did not manifest the same largeness of spirit as did Zurich," writes a modern French scholar.[86] In the periodicals and medical journals of the late 1860s and early 1870s are many traces of the strong opposition to the government's decision to allow women into the Ecole de Médecine. At the time of Putnam's entrance, for example, Dr. Henri Montanier, in a widely commented upon article, wrote that nature had dictated a far different role for women than the brutalizing practice of medicine. "She is destined above all to be a spouse, a mother," he argued, "and to live a private life [*vivre dans l'interieur*]." To be a doctor and enter the harsh world outside the home, he warned, a woman must destroy her essential traits of tenderness, modesty, and gentility. Women might have the same ability as men and the law might make the study of medicine possible, but "as a man, as a moralist, as a philosopher" he pleaded that parents protect their daughters from such a career.[87] More than in Britain or America, as Mary Putnam had told her mother, opposition to women in France was based on moral grounds, on fears of changes in women's nature, rather than on doubts about their physical or intellectual capacity.

By 1873, when the Russian women arrived in Paris, the debate was at a fever pitch. After questioning a large number of students about the presence of women in medical classes, a Paris physician reported that they had all responded with disgust. The women involved, he charged, were losing "all their grace, all their charm, all that was attractive in their sex."[88] Another doctor concluded a long tirade against the women medical students with the sentence: "By the laws of physiology, the woman doctor is a . . . hermaphrodite or without sex, in any case a monster."[89] Still another pointed to the clear moral danger of promiscuity when women were placed in the same lecture halls and clinics as men.[90] Even in America, the "land of absolute liberty," said a French social science encyclopedia in 1874, the study of medicine by women was encountering very serious difficulties. Citing the student protests and demonstrations in Philadelphia, the writer claimed that such disorders, while regrettable, could not be avoided so long as women kept up their senseless campaign to become doctors.[91]

Even though it was foreign women, rather than native French women, who made up the great majority of those studying in Paris, there was clearly fear that they were but the entering wedge of a larger movement. It was, in fact, extremely difficult for a French woman to qualify for study in medicine. While foreign women were allowed to substitute the equivalent of a lycée education to gain admission—Mary Putnam, for example, used her professional degrees from Philadelphia and New York to satisfy the requirement—French women, like the native women of Switzerland, had almost no opportunity to prepare in their own country for university study.[92] Not until 1880 did France create a system of public secondary schools for girls, and even then, according to a historian of French universities, there was "fairly stiff" opposition to allowing women into the universities. "French women," he writes, "were far slower than foreigners to embrace so unfeminine a career as medicine."[93]

## A New Beginning

The waves of foreign women who descended on Zurich and Paris in the decade after 1864 marked the beginning of the end of continental resistance to women in medicine. By 1874, more than 150 women had registered for medical study in the universities of Switzerland and France. The great majority of them were Russian, but their ranks included seven Americans, six Englishwomen, four Germans, and two each from Serbia, Hungary, and Russian Poland.[94] What is striking about these women is that they became the leaders of a whole generation of women physicians in Europe and America. In England, the pioneer physicians who established the right of women to practice medicine—Elizabeth Garrett, Elizabeth Morgan, Louise Atkins, as well as Sophia Jex-Blake and Edith Pechey—all took their medical degrees in Paris, Zurich, or Bern. The German pioneers, Franziska Tiburtius and Emilie Lehmus, likewise studied in Zurich in the early 1870s. Nadezhda Suslova and Maria Bokova became legends among the young women of Russia. In the United States, Mary Putnam and Susan Dimock stood at the forefront of the American profession. Of Putnam, William Osler said that few men of her generation could match her preparation in medicine.[95] When Dimock returned to Boston, Zakrzewska wrote that "it is not the Republic of America which has given the proof that 'science has no sex' . . . it is the Republic of Switzerland which has verified this maxim."[96] Until at least the 1880s, most of the women doctors of Europe held diplomas from Swiss universities.[97]

Other nations followed the example of Switzerland and France. Sweden opened the study of medicine to women in 1870, but eighteen years would pass before Karolina Widerström became the first to complete her studies at the Karolinska Institute. A Dutch woman enrolled at Groningen in 1871, but several years elapsed before other women were able to satisfy the requirements for admission in medicine. At the University of Copenhagen in Denmark, two women overcame faculty opposition to enroll in medicine in 1877. In Italy, where historically women had had free access to the universities, a Russian, Ernestine Paper, who had studied in Zurich, became the first woman to graduate in medicine in united Italy in 1877. Still other European nations began to admit women in the 1880s—Belgium in 1882, Norway in 1884, Spain and Portugal in 1889.[98] In all these countries, except Belgium, the study of medicine by foreign women was rare, chiefly because of the lack of familiarity with their languages.

The women's migration to Switzerland and France was heaviest from those countries that were slowest to give women equal treatment in medical education—Russia, Germany, Austria, Britain, and, at a distance, the United States. The Russian government established a four-year medical program for women at the Medical-Surgical Academy in St. Petersburg in 1872 but restricted its teaching to obstetrics, gynecology, and children's diseases. During the course of the 1870s, the program gave promise of developing into a full-scale medical school, only to be closed in 1882 after the assassination of the Tsar.[99] In Germany and Austria, despite the close ties between their medical faculties and those in Zurich and Bern, the political and social climate remained chilly toward women's aspirations in medicine. Franziska Tiburtius, who was among the earliest German students in Zurich, said that "even to apply [to a German medical school] would have seemed absurd and ridiculous."[100] Similarly, in Great Britain, even after the opening of a women's medical college in London in 1874, the established universities did not weaken in their opposition to women students. "The real solution of the difficulty," Elizabeth Garrett wrote to the *Times*, "will be found in Englishwomen seeking abroad that which is at present denied to them in their own country."[101]

But the decision to study abroad was not easily taken. A woman going abroad faced the same trials and vexations that men encountered—the hazards and expense of an overseas voyage, or perhaps a weeks-long journey by wagon or sleigh to a railhead in rural Russia; the costs of tuition, room, board, and books; the perplexity of an entirely different educational system; the difficulty of learning and working in an unfamiliar language; the higher standards and demanding medical examinations of Western Europe; the loneliness of life spent largely alone in a foreign country, and more besides. Women students abroad were much younger than their male counterparts, who often left home only for postgraduate education, some-times after practicing medicine for several years. A woman, too, had often to convince her family that it was not totally senseless for her to become a doctor, much less journey to a foreign land, or else cut herself off from family support as did so many of the Russian women. There was deep concern also for the safety and well-being of a young woman alone on a continent where few women went unchaperoned to public places. A returning male doctor warned Americans in 1880 against taking their wives on study tours to Europe, for they would have to leave them alone a great deal "in a place where ladies do not walk or shop unattended."[102]

The events at Zurich and Paris opened a safety valve for many women who wanted to become physicians. As Russia, Germany, Britain, the United States, and other countries alternately tightened or loosened controls over women's study, the flow of women to these and other pioneer centers waxed and waned. Russia, in par-ticularly, followed an unsteady course in its policies toward women in medicine, but other nations wavered as well in the amount of hope they offered women intent on medical study. In Britain and the United States, where women's medical schools were the principal means of educating women doctors, only those driven by ambition to prepare themselves as well or better than men made the difficult and costly decision to study abroad. The most prestigious of British and American universities, with few exceptions, continued to bar women until the First World War. So it is no surprise that the steady stream of foreign women studying medicine in Switzerland and France continued in the years after 1874, swelled in the late 1880s and 1890s as Russia and Germany faced crises in their policies to-ward women, and finally became a torrent after 1905 when Russia shut down virtually all domestic opportunities for women to study medicine.

# 3 *The Great Migration*

The women returning home from Zurich and Paris were fired with fresh confidence. A new respect greeted them in even conservative bastions. Mary Putnam, for example, was quickly allowed into the county medical society of New York, the second woman after Elizabeth Blackwell, while Susan Dimock won a standing in the Boston profession that had eluded her predecessors.[1] In Great Britain, Elizabeth Garrett, on her return from Paris, ran for election to the London School Board, conducted a dispensary, and helped found a medical school for women, which she would eventually lead.[2] The German pioneers, Franziska Tiburtius and Emilie Lehmus, both graduates of Zurich, were able, despite the deep hostility of their countrymen, to open a popular clinic for women in Berlin.[3] Almost all of the European and American pioneers who studied abroad were to serve, by choice or necessity, in special clinics or schools created to meet the needs of women.

The Russian pioneers were also viewed with new respect. Nadezhda Suslova's fame for her Zurich achievement caused the Russian Medical Council, after a period of hesitation, to allow her to take the examinations for foreign doctors and grant her the right to practice in Russia. For a time, she became the best-known woman in the Russian Empire. Subsequently, she would publish a number of articles in physiology, write short stories, and treat the people in her adopted home in the Crimea without payment.[4] Her close friend, Maria Bokova, likewise a heroine to her generation, did further studies in ophthalmology, translated scientific articles into Russian, and did research at the Russian Academy of Medicine. Like Suslova and most of the European pioneers, she married, in her case twice, the second time to the defender of women's right to study medicine, Ivan Sechenov.[5]

Other Russian women were also able to use the medical training they had gained in Zurich or Bern. After being called home by her revolutionary comrades, Vera Figner got a license as a paramedic (*feldsher*) and then as a midwife before setting out to work for the radical cause in rural Russia.[6] Another former student at Zurich, Anna Tomaszewicz, against all odds, won the right to practice as the first woman doctor in Russian Poland.[7] Still another, Vera Liuba-tovich, was called a "miracle worker" for her ministrations to sick neighbors in Tobolsk province in western Siberia, where she was banished for her revolutionary activity.[8]

## After the Pioneers

The success of the first generation to go abroad encouraged others to weigh the benefits of foreign study. Conditions at home were changing only slowly in many countries. The quickening pace of industrialization left ever more women uncertain and insecure about their futures. It was the powerful force of hunger, according to a group of Swiss academic women, that drove the European women's movement of the nineteenth century—"material hunger for bread of those forced out of their home employments and therewith their homes [and] hunger for self-determination and the freedom to work of those from whom the chance to work in a family community had been taken."[9] By the 1870s and 1880s the struggle had enlisted the support of hundreds, sometimes thousands, of women in Europe and America who organized, petitioned, and fought for greater participation in the economic and professional life of their nations.

From the viewpoint of European women, their sisters in the United States seemed to have made the greatest progress. The American example was cited by German, English, and Russian women in arguing for greater opportunities in their own professional and educational lives. "Nowhere on the face of the earth," wrote the translator of a German feminist's study of women's education in Europe,[10]

> [does] woman occupy so elevated a position as [in the United States] . . . nowhere is her inborn right to education more readily and

willingly acknowledged than here; . . . nowhere are more schools, colleges, and universities open to women than here; . . . nowhere has woman found so many chances for employment in consequence of liberal provisions for her education; and . . . nowhere has the maxim "Education is liberation" been proved more conclusively than here.

By the late 1880s, according to the same study, more than half of the students in American secondary schools were girls, compared to 30 percent in Britain, 29 percent in Prussia, and only 10 percent in France. Women accounted furthermore for almost 30 percent of the enrollment in universities, which contrasted sharply with the 11 percent in Britain, 2 percent in France, and none at all in Germany and Austria.[11]

But in medicine American women found both more and less freedom than their contemporaries in Europe. The leading medical colleges of the United States were as firmly closed to women in 1880 as were the universities of Germany and Austria. No American university approached as yet the openness to women of Zurich or Paris. Only the public universities in the western states even purported to accept women on the same basis as men, and a number of them continued to segregate students on the basis of their sex. It was the irregular schools and the schools for women that still educated the vast majority of women doctors trained in the United States. By the time of the census of 1880, 2,432 women could declare themselves to be physicians.[12] No country of Europe, not even Russia, approached this number of legally qualified women physicians.

While admiration was universal among women's groups in Europe for the American achievement, less was said of the schools in which they were educated. "A sort of misty cloud," recalled Franziska Tiburtius, "hung over the apparition of the female doctor in America."[13] Some could simply not understand how so many women could practice medicine when the best universities and most of the regular schools of medicine were closed to them. European women, especially after the opening of Zurich and Paris, remained hopeful that the established universities of their own countries could yet be won to their example. If forced to leave their homelands, almost all of them chose Switzerland or France for study rather than a women's school in America or Britain.

American women who had been abroad kept up a drumbeat of criticism of the level of women's medical education at home. "There have always come forward a much larger number to claim the right to practice," Mary Putnam (now Mary Putnam Jacobi) told the new students of the Woman's Medical College in New York in 1880, "than to crave the privilege of being thoroughly well educated." The "unfortunate majority" of American women doctors, she charged, "have constantly tended to drag the conditions of medical education down to the level of their capacity, or intention to fulfill them."[14] The following year, three well-known women doctors concluded a survey of 430 women practitioners with these thoughts about the further training of women:[15]

> It is very easy to say that women have their own medical schools, and need nothing more, and to ascribe any attempt to obtain entrance into our best universities to a restless ambition to be masculine. So far as our personal knowledge goes, the majority of women students would prefer not to receive all their instruction in mixed classes, but they want the best, and they know that the women's colleges, though deserving great praise for what they have done, cannot, in the nature of things, offer the advantages of institutions which have for years had the best talent of the country at their command.

By the time of this report, a number of leaders of the American profession were ready to lower the remaining barriers to women. The success at Zurich was used by the Boston physicians Henry I. Bowditch, James J. Putnam, and James R. Chadwick to plead for admission of women to Harvard and other private schools. "We have reached the absurd stage," said Chadwick in 1879, "when the burning question is no longer, Shall women be allowed to *practice* medicine? They are practicing it, not by ones or twos, but by hundreds; and the only problem now is, Shall we give them opportunities for the study of medicine before they avail themselves of the already acquired right of practicing it?"[16] Putnam, too, argued publicly for the admission of women at Harvard, citing the "favorable experience" at Zurich.[17]

Such voices were drowned, however, in the general chorus of opposition to women's study. The editor of the influential *Boston Medical and Surgical Journal*, who never missed a chance to ridicule the women's aspirations, went so far as to feature prominently a false report that Zurich was about to abandon its experiment in educating women. "One would hardly ask," he wrote, "for more satisfactory proof of the impropriety of such experiments than the experience of this school."[18] He was answered promptly from Zurich by Edmund Rose, who flatly denied the report and told American readers that after twelve years women "do not cause any great excitement" in Zurich.[19]

Other nations besides the United States remained skeptical of the women's experience in Zurich and Paris. Favorable reports, such as that of the British surgeon Lawson Tait in 1874, were for the most part ignored.[20] The British profession and its allies, despite growing public pressure, managed to keep women out of all medical schools except those established for women. The highly publicized efforts of Jex-Blake and her companions to gain acceptance at Edinburgh had failed. Women were admitted to no British hospitals except their own; they were excluded from the British Medical Association; they were not allowed to participate in the International Medical Congress in London in 1881; and only twenty-six of them, almost all with foreign degrees, were able to gain recognition as registered practitioners by 1882.[21]

In Germany and Austria, a shrill debate over women's capacity for medicine sounded throughout the 1870s and 1880s. Here and there a woman was admitted to medical classes as an auditor, but the climate for medical women was chilly and forbidding.[22] The Zurich graduates Tiburtius and Lehmus were for fifteen years the only women physicians able to practice in Berlin. "The German is the only and the last great nation of culture," wrote the feminist Helene Lange in 1890, "which leaves its women under the oppression of medieval fetters, keeping the institutions of higher learning closed against them."[23]

Farther east, the Russian government's courses in obstetrics and women's and children's diseases for women, opened with great fanfare in 1872, were suddenly closed a decade later. Nearly a thousand women had studied in these courses and many graduates were already working in hospitals, clinics, *zemstvos* (institutions of local government in rural Russia), and private practice.[24] The need for doctors in Russia was still acute and thousands of young women had had their interest whetted by the courses and the earlier migration to Switzerland. It was again Russian women who would lead the second wave of women to go abroad to the medical schools of France and Switzerland.

So it was that a stream of new migrants, dismayed by conditions at home, followed in the steps of the pioneers at Zurich and Paris. A century later it is hard to visualize the teeming colonies of foreign women who for the next forty years poured into the comfortable old Wohnhäuser in the Oberstrass in Zurich and the crowded student quarters of Bern, Paris, and Geneva. Some stayed only a semester or two; others stayed three or four years; still others completed the entire medical course and wrote a doctoral thesis for the medical degree. A number of them had had some medical training at home or were able to complete their degrees later in their own countries.

The stream of women to France and Switzerland grew heavier toward the end of the century as conditions in Eastern Europe became critical, and reached floodtide in the early years of the twentieth century. In all, on the basis of available evidence, it can be reliably estimated that well over ten thousand individual women, three-fourths of them from the Russian Empire, took some medical training in Switzerland or France in the half-century before 1914. They accounted for a large proportion of all European women with medical experience before World War I. At least a quarter of them held medical degrees from Swiss or French universities. By the early years of the twentieth century the medical enrollment of women in tiny Switzerland alone would exceed that of the 150 medical schools of all kinds in the United States (Table 1).[25]

*Table 1.* Medical enrollment of women in Switzerland, France, and the United States, 1900–1910

| Country | 1900 | 1906 | 1910 |
|---|---|---|---|
| Switzerland | 554 | 1,181 | 753 |
| France | 340 | 454 | 802 |
| United States | 1,467 | 895 | 707 |

*Sources:* For Switzerland, Eidgenössisches Statistisches Amt, *Schweizerische Hochschulstatistik, 1890–1935,* p. 54; for France, *Bulletin administratif du Ministère de l'Instruction Publique,* 1900–01, 1906–07, 1910–11; for the United States, *Reports of the Commissioner of Education* for appropriate years. The U.S. figure for 1910 is a handcount of enrollments in the 1909–10 report of the Commissioner (vol. 2, pp. 1058–1064) and differs from that given by other scholars. It includes 134 homeopathic students.

## The Opening of Bern

After the Russian *ukase* of 1873 the first wave of female migration to the medical school at Zurich had been broken. The enrollment of women remained under 25 for the next decade. American and German women were now prominent among those who came to Zurich (Table 2). By the fall of 1883, 23 American women had registered for formal medical study, including such future physicians as Ellen Powers, Adeline Whitney, Josephine Kendall, Mary Almira Smith, Harriet Lothrop, Kate Woodhull, Elizabeth Bigelow, and Marie Mergler. Several of them gained distinction in their work abroad. Ellen Powers, for example, was chosen by the psychiatrist August Forel to work as an intern in his mental hospital, while Mary Almira Smith got one of the most sought-after student positions in the medical school as an assistant to the surgeon Edmund Rose.[26] When Smith returned to Boston to take up the post of resident surgeon at the women's hospital in 1880, Marie Zakrzewska said that she was determined "to persuade other educated women to study in Zurich so that we can fill this [city] with such graduates and thus overcome little by little the opposition to co-education."[27]

*Table 2.* National origin of women medical students at Zurich, 1865–1914

| | |
|---|---|
| Russia | 971 |
| Germany | 147 |
| Poland* | 111 |
| United States | 56 |
| Austria | 30 |
| Yugoslavia (Serbia and Croatia) | 28 |
| Hungary | 14 |
| Great Britain | 12 |
| Holland | 7 |

*Source:* Handcount of Matrikel der Universität Zürich, 1833–1933, Staatsarchiv, Zurich.

*Includes only those women who declared their country of origin to be Poland or Russian-Poland. The actual figure is higher.

In the meantime, the Russian students at Zurich had begun their exile in Bern, Geneva, and Paris. In Bern, twenty of the Russian women were enrolled in medicine in the fall of 1873. Unlike Zurich, the shock of change came swiftly as women suddenly occupied a sixth of the places in the school of medicine. There had been rumors throughout the summer that a hundred Russian women would descend on the provincial capital. The students held a meeting in July to protest the threatened invasion. In a letter to the Academic Senate they charged that there was too little space in the clinical institutes and not enough teaching material for so many students. "Too generous an attitude toward foreigners," they warned, "would endanger the study of the native students."[28]

The authorities at Bern overrode the student opposition, however, to admit the women provisionally. Since several women, including three Russians and a Swiss-Columbian woman, had already matriculated in the preceding two years, there was precedent for the university's action.[29] As in Zurich, the admission of women enjoyed wide support among the faculty and educational officials of the canton. Such leading medical professors as the surgeon Theodor Kocher and the pathologist Theodor Langhans, as well as the political economist Hans von Scheel, were well disposed toward the female students.[30] Spokesmen for the university, as had happened in Zurich, described the influx of women students as an "experiment" that now claimed the attention of the entire academic community.[31]

The courageous Scheel, elected rector in 1873, devoted his entire inaugural address in November to the question of women's study. The behavior of faculty members and students toward the women, he began, would have serious consequences not only for the university but for the expansion of women's opportunities throughout the industrial world. Carefully he explained that the familiar household economy of Europe, which had provided women as well as men with important social roles for hundreds of years, was fast disappearing. No longer was clothing spun and woven at home; no more were candles, soap, and a thousand daily necessities produced within the household. Women were marrying later in life; more of their lives was spent in supporting themselves outside the family. Above all, they needed education to prepare themselves for a world that was changing. While women were now welcome to fill many jobs in industry, commerce, and teaching, they were still barred from the higher professions. "If women can be kings and workers the same as men," he said, "why not physicians, judges, and officials?" To the argument of the medical students that women were taking up scarce space and displacing "real" students, Scheel replied simply that their case rested on an unallowable premise, namely, "that women's study is less justified than that of men." Nor would he accept the argument that the women's case was weakened by their being foreigners. "Since all our universities have a cosmopolitan character for their own welfare, insofar as they admit male foreigners, how can they then close their doors to women foreigners?"[32] It was a remarkable performance, and his unflinching stand in behalf of women's study helped set the tone for the rapid growth of female enrollment at Bern in the years ahead.

The band of Russian women was joined by a smaller number of women from Germany, Britain, America, and Eastern Europe. The number of women medical students reached 38 in the winter of 1874, leveled off in the next decade, and then rose steadily again to 95 in the winter term of 1891. By this time women accounted for 25 percent of the medical enrollment at Bern, which had surpassed Zurich in its appeal to foreign women. A total of 347 women had studied medicine in Bern and 97 had earned their degrees.[33] Among the Russian women who finished their degrees in these years was Fanny Berlinerblau, a close friend of Franziska Tiburtius in Zurich, who came to America following her graduation and became chief surgeon at the New England Hospital for Women and Children.[34] Nine British women finished their studies in Bern, including such well-known leaders as Jex-Blake, Edith Pechey, and Ann Clark.[35] Jex-Blake later commented on "the thoroughly wholesome indifference" with which women students were treated in Bern compared to Great Britain.[36] Fewer American women came to Bern than to Zurich; only the names of Caroline Davis, Annie Kriemont, and Ida Hoff, all of New York, can be found in the early matriculation records.[37]

The first strong reactions against the foreign students at Bern came in the early 1880s. As in Zurich, the clannishness of the Russian women, their dress and manners, and their interest in radical politics set them off sharply from other students and townspeople. Students were particularly upset by their aggressive competition for favorable laboratory and classroom places. "A cancer on our university" read the headline over a letter from several newspaper readers in 1883, who attacked the "unsuitable student elements" in the medical school.[38] A Swiss woman student recalled that "the hordes of Russian women struck us as foreign, strange, disquieting, and often unpleasant."[39] Friendships between Swiss and foreign students were rare, and tensions often ran high. In 1885 the medical students sent a petition to the cantonal government asking that those without a Swiss diploma or its equivalent be barred from matriculation. But officials of the canton, like those at the university, were unshaken by the student protests. Later, as the number of Russian students rose dramatically, the cries of protest grew louder. The Bern press derided the Russian women as "hyenas of the Revolution," and "seductresses of youth" and their student communities as an "underworld of sickly, half-educated, and uncontrolled creatures."[40] Again, however, the authorities held firm and refused to restrict the numbers of foreign students.

It is remarkable that so many of the political and academic leaders of Switzerland supported the cause of women's higher education so strongly at a time when much of the world excluded women completely or partially from the best education available to men. That most of these women were foreigners and bearers of an unfamiliar culture and ideas makes the achievement even more impressive. A growing proportion of the Russian women were Jews, severely restricted from university attendance at home. After 1886, a strict quota on the number of Jews allowed to study in secondary schools and universities had been instituted in Russia. One careful student of the Russian emigration to Switzerland estimates that by the early twentieth century at least 60 percent of the women were Jewish.[41] It may well have been higher. Pogroms against Jews increased the number of those coming west in 1903, 1904, and especially 1905. Some critics of the liberal Swiss policies toward women and foreigners argued that it was only the bourgeois greed of the Swiss for the money spent by students and the greed of the professors for more tuition payments that made them so open, but these financial incentives clearly existed also in Germany, Britain, and America. In the case of those responsible for university policy at Bern and Zurich, in any case, a certain amount of liberal idealism must clearly be assigned to their actions.

## Geneva and Lausanne

A similar breadth of view characterized the leadership in Geneva and later in Lausanne. At Geneva, which opened its medical school in 1876, two remarkable men, the Polish-born anatomist Sigismund Laskowski and the liberal pathologist Moritz Schiff—both veterans of earlier revolutionary movements—became champions of women's education and the international character of the student body.[42] The radical party in Geneva strongly supported the politics of university expansion and the opening of the university to women and foreigners. Without an international outreach, it was argued on all sides, a dynamic university could not be supported from local interest alone. A distinguished faculty and an international student body would raise the prestige of the city. Said Councilman James Fazy in 1872, in putting the case for a medical school in Geneva, "Erlangen, Tübingen—cities no more important than Geneva—possess a medical school."[43] Twenty years later, when the young medical school had grown to 161 students, 40 percent of them women, the internist Auguste Eternod expressed the satisfaction of his colleagues: "It is clear that the University of Geneva is not able and does not need to recruit exclusively in our little canton, not even in Switzerland, but must struggle always to become an international university. That role it is already filling, especially vis-à-vis the countries to the east."[44]

As had happened in Zurich and Bern, the great majority of the women students at Geneva were enrolled in medicine. Even before the university was formally opened, the Swiss crusader for women's rights Marie Goegg had asked the Grand Council of Geneva in the name of "the mothers of Geneva" to admit women to medicine and other careers. Geneva, she said, should follow the enlightened policies of Zurich.[45] With strong support from both political and academic authorities, the request was approved. The enrollment of women at Geneva grew only slowly, however, owing to the newness of the university and the proven attractions of the other Swiss universities. Only four women had enrolled in the medical school by 1877, and the number remained under ten for the next decade.[46] Then, however, Geneva's appeal to women seeking an opportunity in medicine began to rise. By the turn of the century the female enrollment in medicine at Geneva had overtaken its Swiss rivals and soon left them far behind. As in Zurich and Bern, women from the Russian Empire and Eastern Europe accounted for a large proportion of the students from abroad. In the summer semester of 1900, for example, 107 women were matriculated in medicine as "Russian," compared to only a sprinkling of women from Germany, Italy, Britain, and the United States.[47] Many of those classified as Russian were, in fact, Poles, Armenians, Ukrainians, or Georgians.[48]

Geneva became a favorite destination for the women of Eastern Europe and Russia. Most of them lived together in small communes, had meager resources, and were endlessly active in radical politics. On Chaim Weizmann, who was then teaching in Geneva, they made an impression of being "underfed, stunted, nervous and sometimes bitter—an easy prey to revolutionary propagandists."[49] Nowhere, according to a modern historian, were the ties between students and emigré politicians so close as in "the little Russia" of Geneva.[50] Townspeople were concerned that the crowds of loud, boisterous, poorly dressed students on the streets were endangering the profitable tourist trade. Geneva newspapers wrote constantly of the "Russian invasion" and the "rupture of equilibrium" in the city.[51] A writer for *La Tribune* satirized the behavior of these "pitiable students" who felt "obliged to exercise their eloquence in all the little cafés."[52] By the early years of the twentieth century, concerned Swiss students had organized a campaign to restrict the number of foreigners in the university. As the pressures mounted, a new regulation requiring Russian medical students to meet standards of admission equivalent to those of the Swiss was passed, but sterner measures were beaten back.[53]

Meanwhile, another medical school was opened in French Switzerland. The University of Lausanne, created in 1890, was coeducational from its beginning.[54] Several women, in fact, had already begun the study of medicine in the academy that preceded the university. Within a decade nearly a hundred foreign women were studying medicine in the new university, and by 1902 their number exceeded the male enrollment in the medical school.[55] The early students won the esteem of influential professors, who defended them against the attacks made familiar in other Swiss universities. In 1899, they bestowed on a Russian woman the coveted Cérenville prize for the best original work in anatomy, physiology, or pathology. Other women were likewise recognized by the faculty, and several won highly competitive posts for internships and assistant positions in the clinics and laboratories of Lausanne.[56]

By 1900, Switzerland was educating more women doctors than the rest of Europe combined (Table 3). The last Swiss holdout, the conservative University of Basel, admitted a Swiss woman in 1890 but continued to hold the line against foreign women lacking a Swiss high school diploma.[57] Not until 1906 did foreign women begin to appear in the official statistics of Basel. The other four medical schools, by now accustomed to foreigners and women in their midst, enrolled 554 women in 1900.[58] Since 1867, when Suslova had first matriculated, the Swiss faculties had enrolled nearly two thousand women in medicine. Several hundred additional women had audited medical classes, a common European practice. All but three or four hundred of the registered women had come from nations under Russian control, although the study by non-Russians was significant beyond their numbers. Those from Germany, for example, accounted for the vast majority of all female physicians in that country until the early years of the twentieth century. The American women who studied in Switzerland, on the other hand, numbered less than a hundred, a small fraction of the women physicians in America, but they were among the best educated of women doctors in the nine-

*Table 3.*  Women medical students in Switzerland, 1870–1914

| | |
|---|---|
| 1870 | 14 |
| 1880 | 54 |
| 1890 | 156 |
| 1900 | 554 |
| 1906 | 1,181 |
| 1910 | 753 |
| 1914 | 499 |

*Sources:* Matrikel der Universität Zürich, Staatsarchiv Zurich; Barbara Bachmann and Elke Bradenahl, "Medizinstudium von Frauen in Bern, 1871–1914" (dissertation, University of Bern, 1990), p. 18; H. Henke, *Statistik der Universität Zurich in den ersten fünfzig Jahren ihres Bestehens* (Zurich: Zurcher and Furrer, 1883), p. 52; Eidgenössisches Statistisches Amt, *Schweizerische Hochschulstatistik 1890–1935*, p. 54; Marie Goegg, "Switzerland," *The Woman Question in Europe*, ed. Theodore Stanton (New York and London: G. P. Putnam's Sons, 1884), p. 387.

teenth century.[59] As late as 1897, American women in Zurich were publishing a guide for those who wished to study there. They advised that the normal course in medicine was five and a half years of "very severe labor"; that the university accepted an American college diploma in lieu of an entrance examination; that fees amounted to around seventy dollars a year; and that "no woman should come to Zurich . . . unless she has not only a reading but a speaking knowledge of German."[60]


## The Fight for the Internship in France

Meanwhile, in France, the women who followed in the footsteps of the pioneers of the sixties encountered new problems. Their numbers had begun to rise in the 1870s and then jumped dramatically in the 1880s and 1890s. In Paris alone the number of women in medicine had increased from 18 in 1873 to 37 in 1880 and to 114 in 1887. In the earlier years, English and French women outnumbered those who came from the Russian Empire. In 1881, for example, 11 Englishwomen were studying medicine along with 10 women from France, 9 from Russia, and 5 from the United States.[61] With the closing of the women's schools in Russia, however, and the stringent new quotas on Jewish study after 1886, the proportion of Russian and Polish women rose steadily. By 1887, 70 Russian and 20 Polish women were studying medicine in Paris, along with 12 women from France, 8 from Britain, and a scattering from other countries.[62] As the century ended, 340 women were enrolled in French medical schools, about half of them from areas ruled by Russia, the rest largely from France itself. A majority of the women were found in Paris, with clusters at the other six schools in Montpellier, Nancy, Lyon, Toulouse, Lille, and Bordeaux.[63]

But a major battle was necessary before women were allowed to compete for the highly valued opportunity to do clinical work in the Parisian hospitals. The competition for places to do supervised hospital work during medical study (externship) and later as full-time residents of the hospital (internship) was at the heart of the French system of medical education. Only those who served as both extern and intern had full access to a career in hospital or university life.[64] Successful specialists in Paris and other large cities were all graduates of the internship program. Only a minority of all medical students could be accommodated in the hospital programs, however, so admission had to be strictly controlled through a system of rigid competition (*le concours*).

Since the time of Madeleine Brès, women had been systematically excluded from that competition. Women students staged a series of protests against this discrimination throughout the 1870s.[65] Particularly effective were the efforts of Blanche Edwards, a French woman whose father was an English physician living in France. She and her father made dozens of visits to public officials, wrote countless letters, and lobbied the medical faculty for an opening of the competition to women. Edwards had been initially discouraged from entering medicine at all by the dean of the medical faculty, Alfred Vulpian, a leading pathologist, who had told her "that a woman's role was to create a home and devote herself to her husband and children."[66] In 1881, however, the Supervisory Council (Conseil de Surveillance) responsible for the examinations relented and decided to admit Edwards and another woman, Augusta Klumpke, to the extern examinations. But the carefully worded statement of the Council suggested that the decision applied only to the externship and not to the more closely guarded competition for internships.[67]

Klumpke and Edwards would play crucial roles in the final opening of the Paris hospitals to women. Klumpke, the daughter of an American woman living in Paris, had been influenced to study medicine by the success of Madeleine Brès.[68] She and Edwards had both been admitted to the medical school in 1878. As was the custom in polite French society, both were escorted each day to the lecture hall or clinic by a relative or friend, and then, by Dean Vulpian's order, they were accompanied by the professor into the building. Each time they entered a classroom in the first few weeks, according to Edwards's biographer, they were greeted by shouts, invective, and sometimes bits of paper and confetti.[69] Clearly, they were regarded as more vulnerable to ridicule than the close-knit group of Russian women, whom the male students largely ignored. After a time, the daily tumult subsided and their studies proceeded without interruption. By 1882, they had completed four years of study and were preparing for the extern examinations. Both passed over this hurdle with high rankings, despite a hostile atmosphere in the examination room, and then entered into limited hospital service. Next came the much higher hurdle of seeking to compete for the internship positions that lay at the peak of French clinical education. A formal request from Klumpke and Edwards, citing the regulation that externs could apply after two years, was abruptly denied in 1884. The Supervisory Council, which was unsympathetic to the women's ambition, was supported in its action by ninety former interns, all demanding that women be excluded from the competition. The medical society of the hospitals, too, meeting in several extraordinary sessions, agreed with the Council's decision.[70]

A battle royal followed that consumed the attention of the Parisian medical and political world. Blanche Edwards again led the fight to overturn the decision. Students and faculty members were quickly polarized into Blanchist and Antiblanchist factions. Politicians and public figures joined in the debate. Edwards was burned in effigy on the Boulevard Saint-Michel near the school of medicine. Forty members of the medical faculty, including Jean Charcot, signed a petition supporting the women. Opponents charged that it was unthinkable to imagine a woman residing in the hospital, sleeping in her clothes as male interns did, or catheterizing a male patient or performing a rectal examination.[71]

The medical journals were filled with hostile articles and editorials. "Women have no more place in an interns' room than in an officers' mess," trumpeted *La France Médicale*. "If they want to abuse [our hospitality]," said another writer, they can go to America, "the country of eccentricity and humbug, where they would never have to leave."[72] In the *Revue Scientifique*, an author drew a parallel between a woman in combat and a woman intern facing the bloody emergencies of a hospital. The latter, he said, "would be the same as a female soldier."[73] Old arguments about women's emotionalism and physiological weakness were again raised, as well as the effect of their becoming doctors on the homes and families of France. Supportive voices were heard as well, including that of the physiologist Paul Bert, the reform-minded minister of education following the French defeat of 1870. It was now too late, said Bert, to raise the old arguments about women's capacity; they were already studying medicine and many of the arguments had been proved wanting. "Professional liberty carries with it the freedom to be educated," he wrote, "and it is this . . . that the women students are asking for" in their petition.[74]

Bert's intervention was critical. On 2 February 1885 the city council of Paris, in an unusual step, imposed on the city's hospitals the
requirement that women be allowed to compete for the internship.[75] With this action, Augusta Klumpke became the first woman
to win the coveted appointment as intern, followed by Blanche Edwards. Klumpke's presence in the Paris hospitals brought a new flood
of public interest. A feature story in *Figaro* described the young
woman as "blond-haired and blue-eyed, with an intelligent look,
pale-complexioned, and of striking countenance." Asked for her
reactions to life in the hospital, the American replied simply: "Don't
speak of me; I only demand one thing, to be forgotten now . . .
Medicine captivates me. I wish to devote myself entirely to it. I hope
I will be of credit in later years and my name be forgotten."[76] Two
years after beginning her internship, she married the noted neurologist Jules Déjerine, with whom she collaborated on a classic study
of the anatomy of the central nervous system. Her own paper on
injuries to the brachial plexus was awarded the prize of the Academy
of Medicine in 1886.[77]

Blanche Edwards would serve her internship in a maternity hospital and become a pioneer in gynecological surgery. More than
Klumpke, she encountered coolness and hostility from her hospital
colleagues. Both women were told that they were not welcome in
the interns' quarters.[78] A number of the professors, however, were
civil and some were friendly. The venerable Charcot was impressed
by Edwards's work in his clinic. After presiding at the defense of her
thesis, he admitted that he had not previously imagined that a
woman could be a successful physician. "You are among the best,"
he told her, "you have passed your examinations in a particularly
brilliant way. Nevertheless, I [still] do not see very clearly the justification of such conscientious labors. What do you propose to do?"
Edwards responded simply that she proposed to take care of sick
people but would devote herself particularly to the health of women
and children.[79]

In spite of the success of Klumpke and Edwards, few women were
able to follow in their footsteps. Between 1886 and 1908, only seven
other women were named as interns in the hospitals of Paris, while
six were designated as alternates.[80] The social and professional resistance to the image of women immersed in the blood and gore of
the hospital limited sharply the numbers reaching the internship.

Foreign women, in any case, were less interested in the internship than French women since it did not help them to meet qualifications at home.

By century's end, France was second only to Switzerland in its openness to women medical students. Despite the lingering and often sharp opposition to women's study and the strong resistance to women in hospitals, the normal applicant to medical school met few obstacles. Paris had been followed by Montpellier, which admitted the Scotswoman Agnes McLaren in 1875, then by Bordeaux in 1884, and finally by the remaining medical schools of France[81] (Table 4). Coeducation in medicine was no longer questioned, and no serious movement to establish separate schools arose. Public opinion throughout the country was turning steadily in favor of women doctors. Some medical teachers who had earlier opposed training for women, such as Ernest Legouvé in Paris, changed their minds.[82] Others were now more willing to speak out in behalf of medical coeducation. "All I have seen of the woman medical student," said the physiologist Charles Richet in 1897, "fills me with admiration."[83] And in Bordeaux, about the same time, a professor named Morache

*Table 4.* Women medical students in France, 1870–1913

| | |
|---|---|
| 1870 | 4 |
| 1880 | 37 |
| 1890 | 120 |
| 1900 | 340 |
| 1902 | 312 |
| 1904 | 366 |
| 1906 | 454 |
| 1908 | 558 |
| 1910 | 802 |
| 1912 | 865 |
| 1914 | 869 |

*Sources:* Caroline Schultze, *La femme-médecin au XIX^c siècle* (Paris: Librairie Ollier-Henry, 1888), p. 15; *Bulletin administratif du Ministère de l'Instruction Publique,* 1914.

was quoted as saying: "For our part we have known and do know women doctors . . . as distinguished by their eminently feminine qualities as by their intelligence, by their knowledge without pedantry and their compassionate heart for all suffering. All these qualities and virtues are found united in them and live in the most perfect harmony."[84]

The number of women practicing medicine in France remained small. According to a contemporary account, only 87 women were in active practice in the year 1900.[85] Most were limited to women's and children's practice, some were school physicians, and a few were beginning to specialize in such fields as ophthalmology. Of the more than 1,000 women from all countries who studied medicine in France before 1900, only 208 had completed their work for the medical degree.[86] About one-fourth of the medical graduates were married at the time of a survey in 1888.[87]

## Floodtide

The opening of medical schools in other countries by 1900 might have been expected to reduce the lure of France and Switzerland. The new Johns Hopkins University School of Medicine was opened to women in 1893 and influenced other medical colleges in the United States and Canada toward coeducation. The proportion of women being educated with men in medicine jumped from 40 to 70 percent in the United States between 1890 and 1900.[88] In Britain, the universities of Scotland and a number of regional medical schools were also accepting women by the 1890s. On the continent, Germany and Austria were beginning to move at last to allow women into their medical schools.[89] Meanwhile, in Russia, the women's medical courses had been reopened in 1897. By that year, Russia could count 500 licensed women doctors in its cities and more than 100 in the countryside.[90] Everywhere, it seemed, women could now find the opportunities at home that had earlier driven them into exile abroad. As the opening circular for the Johns Hopkins school described the school's advantages for women: "it will afford to women . . . those opportunities for advanced medical training which they are at present compelled to seek in the great foreign schools of . . . Paris and Switzerland."[91]

But the rising expectations of women, encouraged by these developments, made them less willing to accept continuing discrimination at home. The leading universities of Russia, Great Britain, and Prussia, as well as a number of American universities, still barred the entrance of women into medical school. The flow of German women to Zurich actually increased as the German universities began to relax their ban on women in medicine. A steady trickle of American and British women, too, continued to seek education abroad despite the gains they were making at home. From Eastern Europe the numbers of women coming west for medical study rose steadily around the turn of the century. And in the Russian Empire, large numbers of Jewish and other minority women were still not able to find places in the women's medical schools of their own country.

Then, in 1900, three of the four women's medical schools in Russia were abruptly closed. Beginning in the fall of that year, the numbers of women heading west began to rise dramatically. The chaotic conditions in the Russian Empire caused many Polish and Jewish women, as well as Russians, to seek a secure academic refuge in the West. The student unrest in Russia made officials reluctant to reopen closed schools and universities. No one could be certain that a school would remain open from year to year. As a Russian woman who came to Zurich later recalled:[92]

> At first I thought of Petersburg, where a medical institute for women existed—that would not be so far from Moscow [where her family lived]. The separation from my family, especially my father, would be very hard for me. But he persuaded me away from the idea: the [political] climate in Petersburg was not healthy; study was often interrupted for political reasons, and the danger—rightly or wrongly—of becoming involved in a student demonstration was too great.

The new waves of migration began to inundate the small medical schools of Switzerland and to raise new questions about women's study in France. Swiss schools enrolled 387 foreign women in medicine in the spring of 1900, 533 in the fall, and then the number swelled to 810 in 1902 and 941 in 1905.[93] Women now accounted for 53 percent of all medical enrollment in the country. In France, where more native women were enrolled, the total number of women medical students jumped from 316 in 1900 to 454 in 1905 but still constituted only 7 percent of medical enrollment.[94] Then came the bloody revolution of 1905 in Russia, which sent still more students into exile. At its peak, the number of women studying medicine in Switzerland reached 1,181 in 1906, and in France 869 in 1914.[95] In individual Swiss universities the proportion of foreigners, chiefly women, in medicine was even more spectacular. It reached 68.7 percent in the medical school at Bern, 70.5 percent in Lausanne, and a staggering 77.4 percent in Geneva, compared to 54.5 percent in Zurich.[96]

Not all the women who came west in these years were Russian or Polish. A number of East Europeans, especially Bulgarians, Hungarians, Serbs, Croats, and Romanians, were studying in the Swiss medical schools, especially in Geneva. German and Austrian women favored the German-speaking universities of Zurich and Bern.[97] A sprinkling of Italian, Greek, English, and American women were found in all the Swiss and French schools. Outside the schools of medicine, where Russian women studied in such huge numbers, the proportion of students from other countries was much higher. In the year 1910, for example, nearly a thousand Bulgarians and Germans, most of them male, were studying in Switzerland but mainly in faculties other than medicine.[98] The same pattern obtained in the French universities, except for a much larger number of medical students from Turkey.[99]

The large number of foreigners set off a wave of xenophobia in France and Switzerland. It was less severe in France. The larger universities and cities of that country made it easier to absorb the new student migrants than was the case in Switzerland. In Nancy, for example, where Russian women constituted nearly half of the foreign medical students in 1908, the police kept the Russians under close surveillance but their presence in the city "caused little stir."[100] In Switzerland, however, all the university cities experienced new crises over the demand to restrict foreign students. In Geneva, a movement was launched to levy a special laboratory tax on foreigners, but it was blocked by faculty members and local officials.[101] At Bern, the medical faculty turned down a move to limit foreign women to the clinical departments of the city hospital. "The medical faculty fully supports the complaint of Russian women students," wrote the dean to the cantonal government, "[that] the instruction of medical students requires the use of the nonclinical departments of the city hospital."[102] Everywhere there was talk of a

"Russian invasion" that was bringing disorder and damaging tourism. In Bern, only the staunch leadership of Albert Gobat, the cantonal minister of education, prevented the government from cutting back sharply on the number of foreign women in the university.[103] The rector at Zurich also fought successfully against the idea of a quota. He told critics in 1906 that Russian students paid 57 percent of all the fees at the university. "The accusation that the foreign students bring only costs without contributing anything," he said, "is unfounded."[104] Although requirements were gradually strengthened in all the Swiss universities, the path to medical study remained remarkably free and open.

## The End of an Era

The First World War brought an end to the great migration of foreign women to the medical schools of Switzerland and France. Never again would women journey abroad in such large numbers to study medicine. By this time, most of the nations of Europe and America were admitting women to their own universities and medical schools. Once opened to women, the German universities too had become a center for medical study by foreign women in the years before World War I. Across the world, women doctors had appeared in nearly every country. Special medical schools for women had been launched in India, Japan, Australia, and Latin America. A number of women from China, as well as India, Japan, and Australia, had taken degrees at the Woman's Medical College of Pennsylvania.[105]

The example of Switzerland and France, like the earlier successes in America, was important everywhere in the battle for women's right to study medicine. Both countries led the United States in the medical education of women during much of the decade before the war. Without question, the rapid growth of women practicing medicine in Russia owed much to foreign study. More than 1,600 women were officially counted as physicians in Russia on the eve of the First World War, more than in the rest of Europe combined and second only to the number practicing in the United States.[106] The Swiss universities also provided the only chance for German and Austrian women to prepare themselves in medicine until the very end of the century. When Germany began seriously considering the education of women in medicine, the imperial government made a formal inquiry in Bern concerning the thirty years of Swiss experience in medical coeducation.[107] British and American authorities likewise sent frequent inquiries to Bern or Zurich. The new Johns Hopkins University, for example, asked the medical faculty in Zurich in 1890 for advice about training women in medicine.[108] The example of Zurich was contrasted with that of Harvard by an American woman at the Columbian Exposition of 1893. "How great the contrast between these two great universities," said Professor Helen Webster of Wellesley College:[109]

> The women of the world owe it to the University of Zurich that she has struck the key-note of justice to women, thus making the false note of injustice the more distinctly heard around the world. It is not merely that Zurich teaches women . . . that she has made the women of all the world her debtors . . . She teaches devotion to learning and to science. It is not on her boatcrews, it is not on her trained athletes that she relies for distinction. She does not furnish entertainment for the diversion of her students . . . It is in the achievements of her ablest professors, in the new recruits which she brings to the cause of science, that she crowns her hope . . . Let the women of the world rejoice that opportunities like these are accessible to them.

But the era of Swiss and French dominance in women's medical education was over in 1914. A new generation of women in Europe and America had begun to know opportunities that were not radically different from those of men. The war itself brought new avenues for medical service in all the belligerent countries. The German feminist Marianne Weber wrote during the war of the generational change that had overtaken women in the universities. The first generation, she wrote, had needed to be fighters who sometimes forced their way into the lecture halls. "They had all by strenuous personal efforts forced their entry into the university. They had to break the many barriers, especially the Chinese wall of a thousand-year-old ideal of femininity that limited the choice of women to the needs of the men." They had climbed over barbed wire, she said, and turned their backs on their family traditions. After forcing their way in, they had still found themselves regarded as strange creatures and had tried to conceal their femininity in dress, attitude, and hair. The pioneers had repressed much in their personalities that was soft and youthful; they had needed to be hard and combative; from repeated rejection had come a satisfying kind of fulfillment. Now, however, the way was open and women had real choices. They no longer needed to sacrifice their femininity in making those choices. How to study and prepare for a career and still be a woman, she concluded, was now the main question for many.[110]

But for Russian women, the struggle to create a new life was subordinate to the social turmoil of their country. For more than half a century, the pursuit of medical education by women had been conducted against the background of chaotic change and revolutionary activity. The universities where they studied, both at home and abroad, were consumed by political agitation and anxious tension. The trials of the Russian woman doctor in the years before 1914 deserve special treatment in any account of women's struggle for education in medicine.

# 4 *Women, Medicine, and Revolution in Russia*

"Was there ever such a place as turbulent Russia before the Revolution?" asks Alix Kates Shulman in her introduction to *Five Sisters: Women against the Tsar*. Women of that time and place, she writes, were

> different from all others we have known: more ascetic and idealistic in tone, humbler and tougher . . . [different] from the women of our own, more familiar radical movements, so often forced to choose between playing "helpmate" and remaining separatist. These women [had] ties of consciousness shared neither by the men of their time nor the women of ours. Looking at their pictures one feels they are a singular breed: soulful, serious Russian originals.[1]

The women of no other nation fought so hard for so long against such fearsome odds to learn the arts of healing. Although Swiss and French universities had been open to women since the late 1860s, relatively few Swiss or French women had taken advantage of the chance to learn medicine. Russian women, as we have seen, outnumbered the native women of Switzerland and France in their own universities.[2] When Germany and Austria finally opened their medical schools to women, the Russians outnumbered the German and Austrian women, too, in a number of their schools.[3] The women of Great Britain likewise studied medicine in far smaller numbers than their sisters to the east. Relatively few women in Italy, Spain, Scandinavia, or the Lowlands prepared for medicine before 1914.

Only across the Atlantic were large numbers of women able to study for the medical profession, but the hurdles faced by American women were far lower than those confronting the Russians. Both relied heavily on women's schools but those in Russia were only intermittently open and placed strict limitations on enrollment. Hundreds were turned away from the courses for women—which lacked the legal protections of the British and American schools for women—and were driven into exile abroad.

After the Women's Medical Institute was finally opened in St. Petersburg in 1897, enrollment of women in Russia began to grow rapidly. By 1906 it had reached 1,635 in St. Petersburg alone and women's medical schools were springing up in Odessa, Kiev, Moscow, and other cities. Still, an equal number of women were being turned away for lack of space.[4] By this time, Russia was educating more than twice the number of women doctors being trained in the United States.[5] As the First World War began in 1914, the Russian medical profession could count a higher proportion of women than any other country: 10 percent of its physicians and 43 percent of its medical students were women; nearly three thousand women were practicing medicine.[6] About a thousand more were being graduated each year, in addition to the hundreds completing their studies abroad.

How was it that the women of Russia and its subject nations achieved so much despite the suffocating atmosphere of Imperial Russia? Certainly they shared the same liberating impulses that drove the women of Western Europe and America—an economic revolution that transformed their lives, the movement for broader women's rights, the heritage of Enlightenment and French Revolutionary ideas, a hunger for self-fulfillment—but they broke more completely than Western women with the social and family conventions that bound them to home and hearth. They asserted a kind of independence that came much later to women in Europe and America. "The ideas of individual freedom and equality of women advanced by the nihilists and absorbed by progressive society," writes Ruth Dudgeon,[7]

> developed an inner spiritual freedom in a number of Russian women . . . these women were confident of their equality with men and of their ability to be doctors, lawyers, mathematicians, chemists, historians, or whatever other professions appealed to them. It was this sense of personal worth which gave Russian women the strength to push their demands and to seek the fulfillment of their intellectual strivings in Russia and throughout the European continent . . . for the

majority of women, conflict between the sexes was not perceived as the problem. For most women, the problem was conflict between a reactionary government and progressive society.

The experience of Russian women was different from that of others, too, in the degree of acceptance of their strivings by important segments of the larger society—teachers, physicians, editors, and university officials. Women medical students met repeated encouragement from their professors; the universities themselves petitioned to be allowed to admit them; physicians campaigned to keep women's courses open; and even the organized medical profession supported them at crucial times. The thousands who had gone west were welcomed back by male colleagues and encouraged to continue or complete their education. The German feminist, Käthe Schirmacher, writing in the early years of the twentieth century, described the special characteristics of the women's movement in Russia as "its individuality, its independence of the momentary tendencies of the government, and the companionable cooperation of men and women."[8] "Looking back in my professional life," the physician Elsa Winokurow would write after leaving Russia for Germany, "I must say that an educated woman was shown more comradeship and courtesy from [the men] in Russia than in Germany."[9]

The internal conditions in Russia that propelled the first women to Zurich in the 1860s were unique in the Western world. A near-feudal structure of social relationships was shaken to its core by dramatic political and social upheaval. The humiliating defeat of the Russian armies in the Crimean War brought an agonizing reexamination of the nation's most revered institutions. The liberation of Russia's serfs in 1861 came to a nation already caught in the throes of industrialization; new scientific ideas, especially those of Charles Darwin, swept over the universities and the ranks of the intelligentsia; a heady, optimistic wave of revolutionary expectation made progress and change the key words of the younger generation.[10] The freeing of the serfs and the collapse of the small landowner economy destroyed the lesser nobility and displaced many into the cities. No longer could holders of small and medium-sized lands depend on the labor of others to give them an income. Daughters in these families, often with no hope of marrying, felt themselves to be a burden on their parents.[11] "The fight for existence," wrote a contemporary historian, "spread to a circle of persons who never before had known money troubles." It was now necessary, he said, "to assure the survival of daughters by learning a profession."[12]

Ideas of women's liberation and equality spread like wildfire in the heated intellectual discussions of the early 1860s. Turgenev's use of the term "nihilist" to describe the central figure in *Fathers and Children* was adopted by many of the younger generation. "By rejecting authority and anything resembling it," said a Soviet writer, "nihilism sent on its way the idea of equality of all people without distinction. To nihilism . . . Russia owes the well-known and remarkable fact that in our culturally deprived country, women began, earlier than in most civilized states, their surge toward higher education and equal rights."[13] Committed to radical change, irreverent toward authority, defiant in dress and manner, the Russian "women of the sixties" showed a hardness and determination to achieve their goals that puzzled and often shocked polite circles inside and outside of Russia. Their perseverance in seeking higher education in the face of withering obstacles, especially in science and medicine, astounded their teachers and fellow students. To many, science was the key to modernization and to their own usefulness in a society undergoing change. Not only did they study medicine in unprecedented numbers but Russian women led women of other countries in winning the first doctorates in mathematics, chemistry, zoology, and physiology.[14]

The education of women was the first major reform to emerge from "the self-flagellating atmosphere following the debacle of the Crimean War."[15] The government had acted in the late 1850s to set up a system of secondary or middle schools for girls of all social classes. Girls would now study such subjects as physics, geometry, Russian, and history, as well as such practical skills as sewing and drawing. By the end of the 1860s, 150 of these schools were teaching more than ten thousand students.[16] This reform, Cynthia Whittaker reminds us, "antedated by fifteen years the first public day schools for girls in England and by thirty years the *lycées des demoiselles* in France."[17]

## Higher Education for Women

Women were first noticed in the lecture halls of universities in Russia in 1859. A law student in St. Petersburg later recalled seeing the daughter of a well-known architect in his classes in the fall of 1860. Other women began coming to classes and by the early 1860s they were a "common sight."[18] Since it was not necessary to register to attend classes as an auditor, most professors, in the liberal spirit of the times, made no objection. A wide mixture of students, both male and female, took advantage of the new openness in higher education. One contemporary noted that "We joyfully observed among us many . . . students from the milieus of all classes of our society."[19] Among the women attending lectures in these early years were Nadezhda Suslova and Maria Bokova. The movement to admit women spread quickly beyond St. Petersburg to other universities in Kazan, Kiev, and Kharkov. By 1862, according to a Kiev professor, "a significant part of the lecture hall was filled with short-haired noble-women in blue-tinted glasses." Unlike the situation in St. Petersburg, the women auditors at Kiev were required to submit the written approval of the professor to university authorities before being allowed to attend a class.[20]

The movement entered a new phase in February 1861. A school-teacher from Kharkov, Liudmila Ozhigina, petitioned the Medical-Surgical Academy in St. Petersburg for the right to enroll as a student. She had been attending lectures in anatomy at the University of Kharkov and had been encouraged to continue her studies. Her petition was refused by the president of the Academy but provoked wide discussion in the universities and the public press. Should women be admitted to full degree status, the universities were asked. All the faculty councils across Russia responded favorably except for Moscow and Dorpat.

A commission was then appointed by the Ministry of Education to review the matter. Much of the medical press was supportive of allowing women into the medical schools. A leading newspaper in St. Petersburg argued that women doctors were greatly needed throughout Russia to spread knowledge of health and hygiene and to care for women whose modesty prevented them from seeking medical help.[21] Opposition was strong, however, to the idea of women studying the healing arts. Arguments familiar to women in America and England were put forward about women's physical strength, their monthly menstrual periods, and their natural modesty. The head of the faculty council at Dorpat, for example, dismissed the idea of women doctors abruptly, saying that "the female sex, due to the peculiarities of its construction and mental and emotional traits," was not suited to the study of either anatomy or medicine.[22]

In the meantime, several women were quietly admitted to medical lectures at the Medical-Surgical Academy. One of the first was Suslova, followed by Bokova, Varvara Kashevarova, and Marie Bogdanova. Several members of the medical faculty, especially Ivan Sechenov and Ventseslav Gruber, encouraged the women's unofficial presence in the Academy.[23] Within two years, more than sixty women could be counted in the Academy lectures.[24] Their studies were abruptly ended in 1864, however, when all the women, except for Kashevarova, were ordered out of the Academy. The government's tolerant attitude had been transformed by a series of student demonstrations and strikes in the early 1860s. Women students had sympathized with the protesters and sometimes taken a direct part. Bogdanova, for example, spoke at a public demonstration and urged the students to fight for their rights.[25] The liberal Nikolai Milyutin, who had been sympathetic to the women students, now described them as *"revolutionnaires* in crinoline, who are of all the most fanatical."[26] Women were henceforth banned from the universities both as students and as auditors.

## The Case of Varvara Kashevarova

The ban on women's study, which lasted in medicine until 1872, was responsible for sending the first wave of students to Zurich. Only Varvara Kashevarova, who intended to work among the Moslem women in Orenburg and whose study was supported by military authorities there, was left among the male students at the Medical-Surgical Academy. Bokova and Suslova, who also promised to work among the physician-shunning Moslem women, were denied further study. Kashevarova thus became the first woman to complete her medical education in Russia itself. A Jewish orphan from Belorussia, she had run away from home at age twelve, fallen ill with typhoid fever, and been rescued by hospital workers who found her a home with a retired sea captain in St. Petersburg. She was illiterate until taught to read by a ten-year-old boy in the family. Adopted by still another family, she was occasionally put in the care of an elderly teacher, who fired her ambition to gain an education. At age fifteen she was married to a store-owner twenty years her elder, who prom-

ised to meet her demand that she be given a chance to study. But
she quickly became unhappy at her treatment in her husband's conservative, old-fashioned family. He refused to support her schooling
further, saying "that he himself was unlearned, and a wife must not
be more intelligent than the husband." As quarrels between them
escalated, she made the decision to leave him.[27]

Kashevarova then entered the Midwife Institute in St. Petersburg,
where she finished the two-year course in eight months "with distinction." A chance meeting with an army medical officer led to
further training for a difficult post in Orenburg province giving limited treatment to Bashkir women. Feeling still unprepared, she asked
to study in the Medical-Surgical Academy. The governor-general of
Orenburg, supporting her, said that "the fulfilling of the request of
the midwife Kashevarova [I] consider very useful for the region."[28]

After the ban on women at the Academy, Kashevarova was the
only woman allowed to study medicine in Russia for the next eight
years. "They all looked at her and caught her slightest mistake," she
said of herself, "but she did not remember that they laughed at her
or made her the butt of their jokes."[29] Some of the women students
who had been expelled asked her to withdraw voluntarily as a ges-
ture of solidarity with the women's cause, but she refused.[30] In her
studies, she developed a strong interest in pathology under the influence of Mikhail Rudnev, a student of Virchow's in Berlin who
later became her husband. In 1868 she presented to the Society of
Russian Physicians in St. Petersburg a paper on *endometritis decidualis,*
which was published in both Russian and German journals. Shortly
afterward, she was accepted into membership in the Society. Against
strong resistance she was allowed to take her final examinations in
1868. The result of a long series of examinations in twenty-seven
separate subjects left her near the top of her class. She was given
her diploma, *cum eximia laude,* on 9 December 1868 "to great ap-
plause." A New York medical journal described how her comrades
in the Academy carried her around the room seated in an armchair.
She would later recall her student days as the happiest in her life.[31]

## Medical Courses for Women

At the banquet celebrating Kashevarova's achievement, a number
of the celebratory speeches called for the opening of medical edu-

cation to all women. One of the speeches came from the daughter
of a prominent member of the medical faculty, who made a dramatic
plea for the ending of the ban on women's study.[32] By this time,
Suslova had returned from Zurich with her medical degree and been
enthusiastically received in liberal circles. The physiologist Sechenov,
her former teacher, described Suslova's achievement as a sterling
example to women seeking an education.[33] Her success, as we have
seen, encouraged other women to undertake the long journey to
Zurich.

The years after 1864 had been painful for many Russian women.
Barred from study at home, they faced the wrenching decision of
laying their educational plans aside or making a difficult and expensive trip to study in a foreign country. Women going abroad were
furthermore required to have their father's or husband's permission
to leave their families. A "fictitious marriage" to a willing friend was
sometimes the only recourse for those leaving home. Those who
went abroad in this period were of necessity from enlightened or
privileged families, or else extraordinarily courageous in the pursuit
of their aims. Of the first wave of Russian medical women in Zurich,
according to one analysis, fourteen came from the nobility, twenty-
seven from the privileged classes (clergy, military, free professions),
two definitely from the lower orders of society, and another twenty-
seven were unidentified by class.[34]

The safety valve at Zurich was open only to a minority of those
ambitious to become doctors. A campaign to reopen medical courses
to women in Russia itself began to gather momentum in the wake
of Suslova's success and the graduation of Kashevarova from the
Medical-Surgical Academy. A speech by a well-known feminist
writer, Eugeniia Konradi, to the Congress of Naturalists in early 1868
added to the public's interest in the "woman question." In her remarks, which were read by a sympathetic professor (women were
not allowed on the floor), she used a new tactic in the debate, that
the mothers of Russia needed to be better educated not only for their
own sake but for that of men as well.[35] Shortly thereafter, four
hundred women, many of them prominent, signed a petition to the
rector of the University of St. Petersburg, asking him to open the
lectures and courses to women. They were supported by a number
of the professors, who declared themselves ready to give lectures to
women in history, philosophy, and natural science.[36] More and

more, the question was being asked: Why should women be forced to go to a foreign country to be educated?

The drive toward medical education for women was boosted by growing concern about the activities of the women students in Zurich. Governmental officials were handed reports that the Zurich students were becoming radicalized by their contacts with Russian emigrés in the city. By the early 1870s Zurich had indeed become the center of Russian revolutionary activity abroad.[37] The government felt growing pressure to provide a chance at education at home, where the women could be more easily watched. Even the conservative Minister of Education, Dmitry Tolstoy, was won over to the idea of university courses for women since they "stopped the flow of Russian women into foreign universities."[38] When the ban on women's study in Zurich was finally published in 1873, it contained a promise of new opportunities to study medicine and other subjects in Russia.

The decision to offer medical courses for women was reached in 1872. It followed the government's earlier action in permitting popular lecture courses outside the university in St. Petersburg (the Alarchin courses) in April 1869 and a month later in Moscow (the Lubyanka courses). More than seven hundred women had attended these lectures in the first year.[39] By the early 1870s the climate for women's education had definitely improved. A friend of Peter Lavrov's captured the excitement of the times when he wrote him that "on the street you constantly meet up with young women with notebooks and books, hurrying somewhere with a distracted air."[40] A proposal from professors at the Medical-Surgical Academy to make at least limited medical training available to women was now viewed more sympathetically. They suggested that two kinds of training be offered to women to improve the level of women's care in the country. In addition to a course in midwifery (*povivalnaia babka*), they urged an advanced level of training, four years in length, for women who would be called "learned midwives" (*uchenaia akusherka*). These women would take essentially the same courses and examinations as doctors (*lekar*) and would be able to treat both women's and children's diseases. The proposal was unanimously approved by faculty councils in the universities, some of whom urged a full medical course for the women. After a long delay in the labyrinthine bureaucracy of the education ministry, the plan was forwarded to the Tsar for approval by the liberal-minded Minister of War, Dmitry Milyutin, who had authority over the Medical-Surgical Academy.[41]

The women's medical courses were opened on 1 November 1872. Described as a four-year "experiment," the courses were to be privately financed (a donor had given fifty thousand rubles to support them), kept completely independent of the men's courses, and controlled by extremely tight social regulations. To study, women were required to have the permission of either their parents or husbands; a minimum age of twenty was established (it was seventeen for men); and they had to show financial assets sufficient to cover the whole four years. Their personal lives and appearance were closely scrutinized. Their hair had to be pulled back into a net; they were required to observe Lent and religious holidays; they were forbidden to smoke, to applaud professors, or to walk in the main corridors of the Academy (where the men studied).[42] In all, eighty-nine women passed the entrance examinations to be admitted to the first class.

They were drawn from all ranks of society, more so than the women who went to Zurich. Only four came from noble families, thirty were daughters of officials, one was from a peasant family, one the daughter of a soldier, and six were identified legally as petty bourgeois. A considerable number were Jews who had limited opportunities otherwise for study.[43] The women came from all over European Russia and Russian Poland. Fourteen of them were married and three were widowed. The course of study was hard and the life of these early students was ascetic. They took virtually the same courses as the men and they were taught by the same professors. Some had studied abroad or in the unofficial classes taught privately by Academy professors, but many suffered from their weak preparation for medical study. They lived in constant fear that the "experiment" would be stopped. Money was extremely tight and many relied on charity for their meals. Tea and black bread were sometimes their only nourishment. Some worked at part-time jobs to earn their keep. Twelve of the women died before completing the course, eight of them from tuberculosis and two by suicide.[44]

For the Russian women who could not go abroad, the Academy courses were a godsend. Far more women applied for the limited number of places in the inaugural class than could be accommodated. Enrollment continued to exceed the official limit of seventy in each class as officials found it difficult to choose among the many eager candidates. The women enjoyed the enthusiastic support of the professors, many of whom gave special help to those having trouble. Most professors returned the stipends given them from the collection of student tuition. Especially beloved was the chemist (and composer) Alexander Borodin, who reserved a special room in his laboratory where the women could come to talk about medicine, music, and their future plans. Outside the Academy, police and governmental officials kept up a close watch on the medical women. All requests from the women, even the establishment of their own medical library, were viewed with suspicion. A number of them were called to the offices of the secret police to be questioned about alleged revolutionary activity.[45]

Anna Shabanova was a member of this first group at the Academy. The historian Jeanette Tuve has written sympathetically of her ardent desire to get a medical education, how she became self-supporting at age fifteen, earned a living by tutoring and translating, and attended Helsingfors University in Finland because she could not afford to go to Zurich. For two and a half years she made her own living while following the university lectures in Swedish. In 1873 she returned to St. Petersburg to join the second-year students in the women's medical course. (Others returning from Zurich, Shabanova reported, also enrolled in the courses.) She found the rules entirely too strict for a group of adult women but like others accepted them in the interest of a chance to study at home. After graduating in 1877, she was allowed, despite the rules barring women from military hospitals, to take advanced training in pediatrics at the Nicholas Army Hospital and also to help other women in their clinical work in children's diseases. In time, she became a senior physician at the hospital, published more than forty articles, and wrote a widely used handbook on first aid. By the first decade of the twentieth century she had become a leading figure in the Russian women's movement. On the fiftieth anniversary of her graduation she was honored by the Soviets as a Hero of Labor.[46]

Shabanova was typical of many of the young women who attended the courses at the Academy in the 1870s. Hundreds of women whose situation would not permit them to go abroad vied for the small number of openings in each medical class. Of the 959 women accepted in the first ten years, 700 finished the course. The average age at entrance was 21.8 years. Eighty-four were married or widowed when they began their studies, and nearly 75 percent were married within eight years of leaving the Academy.[47] The majority of them wrote dissertations in the fields of obstetrics, gynecology, or pediatrics, but some studied problems in psychiatry, surgery, and ophthalmology. Five of the women became surgeons, 16 found employment in psychiatry, and the rest were concentrated in general practice for women and children.[48] Of those who graduated, 54 found jobs in clinics and laboratories, 62 served in women's and children's hospitals, and others were employed in *zemstvos*, state hospitals, public health agencies, or private practice.[49]

As the trial period for the courses came to an end in 1876, the experiment was declared a success. No longer was the women's study to be described as "temporary." The course of study itself was renamed Women's Medical Courses in place of the hated "courses for learned midwives." It was also extended in length to five years and made equivalent to the course for men. In order to separate the women's course more completely from that of the men, it was moved to the Nicholas Army Hospital. New funding was also forthcoming from the Ministry of War and the National Medical Council.[50]

Still undecided, however, were the questions of what title the women graduates would receive and what restrictions would be placed on their practice. Their teachers petitioned that the women be accorded the same status and rights as other graduates of the Academy. This request, however, fell afoul of the state bureaucracy and a final decision seemed years in the future.

Outside events now intervened. In 1877 Russia found itself in a devastating war with Turkey. The shortage of doctors and nurses threatened Russia's ability to care for its wounded. Students in their final year at the Academy, as was the custom, were sent to the front as physicians. This time, the women asked to be allowed to serve too. Twenty-five of the fifth-year women volunteered as military doctors, along with twelve from the fourth year, who were inducted as nurses. Twenty of the physicians were sent to the fighting areas, while five served with the Red Cross in the staging areas to the rear. All were certified as having completed a full course of study.[51]

The conditions they found on the battlefield were appalling. Wounded men were left for hours without treatment, and typhus was everywhere rampant. "Many patients are not even placed in tents but only under curtains," wrote Varvara Nekrasova: "In order to get to them, you have to bend down and crawl on your knees from one patient to the next." Some of the women were sexually harassed and others were taunted by officers and men.[52] Women with no previous experience were suddenly performing dozens of amputations; four of them worked as long as eighteen hours per day caring for nine thousand sick and wounded men at Bulgareni. Some succumbed to the immense pressures. One woman doctor hanged herself; three others, including Nekrasova, perished from typhus. Reports of their self-sacrificing behavior had a powerful effect on officials and public alike. The Tsar awarded each of them a highly coveted military decoration. Dostoevsky hailed their "heroic deeds" and said that all Russia set its hopes for spiritual renewal on them.[53]

Yet the returning women had no clear legal right to practice medicine. Those who had stayed behind took their final examinations before a commission of faculty members and special guests from the Medical Council and the military. "With such an abundance of stars, ribbons, and full dress coats," wrote Anna Shabanova, who was taking the examinations, "it was possible to think of this meeting as a gala spectacle; but in reality it was a tribunal court, created to decide the question whether there was to be or not to be women doctors in Russia."[54] The verdict for the moment was negative. Despite outstanding examinations, the women were given only a provisional certificate that they had completed the course and the right to practice as "learned midwives" among women and children. In 1880, however, Tsar Alexander, undoubtedly influenced by what he had personally seen and heard of the women's performance in war, granted them the title of "woman doctor" with the right to practice medicine. Their new insignia permitted them to practice in schools, *zemstvos*, and state institutions, as well as in private practice.

## New Setbacks

By the early 1880s women's education in medicine seemed firmly rooted. The flow of Russian women to the West had been slowed. Hundreds of women were now applying each year to study medicine. A tenth of all the medical students in Russia were now women. One in three of them was Jewish. Other courses of study for women had been opened during the 1870s. It was small wonder that the feminist leader Elena Likhachëva could claim in 1880 that "Russia has out-stripped other countries [in opportunities for women] and Russian women have achieved greater results."[55]

But the early optimism was not warranted. In official circles, a high degree of skepticism still permeated the discussion of women's future in medicine. The Minister of Education, Dmitry Tolstoy, was an unrelenting opponent of any extension of educational opportunities for women. Existing courses, furthermore, rested on only the shakiest of legal foundations. With the assassination of Alexander II in 1881, old fears of student radicalism were swiftly revived. Even before the attack on the Tsar, the government had quietly advised local officials to consult the secret police before hiring a graduate of the Women's Medical Courses.[56] Now a tide of political repression swept over the universities and medical courses. The liberal Minister of War, Dmitry Milyutin, who had made the women's medical opening at the Medical-Surgical Academy possible, was removed from office and replaced by a far more conservative successor.

Opinion was further stirred by the political trials of 1881. Six of the eight women defendants had received medical training or done work in medical institutions. Sofia Perovskaia, for example, who played a key role in the murder of the Tsar, had been trained as a doctor's assistant (*feld'sher*) and had treated wounded men from the war in Turkey; Gesia Gelfman had taken a course in midwifery in Kiev before making her apartment a center for the manufacture of bombs; Elizaveta Kovalskaia had studied medicine in both Zurich and St. Petersburg before her arrest for revolutionary activities. All six were convicted for their part in the assassination: Perovskaia was hanged; Gelfman died in prison; Kovalskaia was exiled; and the others were imprisoned or exiled.[57] A number of the other students who had gone to Zurich or Bern or Paris were likewise active in the revolutionary movement. The "Fritschi" group, for example, named for a rooming house in Zurich, was particularly watched by the police, especially after many of them joined the All-Russian Social Revolutionary organization in 1875. In all, at least twenty-eight of the former medical students in Zurich were considered "first rank criminals" by the police.[58]

Yet the large majority of women medical students, especially those in St. Petersburg, most scholars are agreed, played little part in the revolutionary turbulence of these years. Not more than 10 percent of the women studying in St. Petersburg were involved with the police, and only four were actually convicted of crimes.[59] It made no difference. The first rumors that the medical courses might close came in the fall of 1881. Conflict within the government added to the uncertainty. It was known that the new Tsar, Alexander III, was not sympathetic to the cause of women's education. Milyutin's successor as Minister of War, General P. N. Vannovskii, was likewise unfriendly. He suggested that the women's courses be shifted to a less prominent site in one of the other hospitals in St. Petersburg. The head of the Interior Ministry rejected the suggestion, claiming that Russia already had a surplus of doctors and no longer needed the women's courses. From the Minister of Education came a curt response that he had no medical faculty within his jurisdiction to take responsibility for the courses. As word leaked out, the professors who had been teaching the women tried vainly to find another sponsor for the courses. By the summer of 1882, however, the die was cast and an imperial decree closed down the courses, with the provision that current students (including those accepted for the fall of 1882) would be allowed to finish. The remaining courses for women in other subjects, with few exceptions, were also closed during the 1880s.[60]

The closing of the medical courses came as a shock. Neither teachers nor students had believed that the progress in medical education for women could be undone. In Warsaw, women secretly organized a series of lectures in private homes that reached two hundred students, including Maria Sklodovskaia (later Madame Curie). A new wave of discussions about the place of women in medicine swept over the Russian press and other public forums. Across the Empire, efforts were made to persuade the government to reopen the women's courses. A group of Moscow women undertook to raise money for their support. The sum of seven hundred thousand rubles was raised in Moscow and other cities. From the city government of Odessa came ten thousand rubles; women in Tiflis raised fourteen hundred rubles from a dance evening; the Sabashnikov family in Moscow gave forty thousand rubles; Professor S. P. Botkin left twenty thousand rubles in his estate for the courses; and one widow promised an annual contribution of a thousand rubles. Dozens of newspapers campaigned for a continuation of women's medical education. Medical journals carried articles in favor of their renewal.

The novelist Turgenev wrote that "all the honorable people of Russia, all who love their homeland . . . are behind you in this question."[61] But all these efforts failed. The women physicians were further humiliated in 1883 when the Tsar ordered the reintroduction of the title "learned midwife" for those who had graduated in medicine.

The last students were taught in 1887. For the next ten years no woman was allowed to study medicine in Russia. A new wave of women set out for Zurich, Bern, Paris, and other universities. The number of Jewish emigrées rose steadily as they were increasingly barred from the severely limited educational possibilities available at home. Eugeniia Weintraub of Kiev, for example, went to Zurich in 1884 to study medicine after finding all other possibilities at home closed to her. Subsequently, she studied in Geneva and was arrested at the Russian border on her return for possessing illegal literature.[62] Guidebooks for students wanting to study in Western Europe began to appear.[63] Again the cry was raised that the women studying abroad were being radicalized and alienated from their native land. The government tried unsuccessfully to persuade the Swiss government to accept only students recommended by the Russian embassy.[64]

Efforts were renewed in Russia to get the St. Petersburg Duma to take responsibility for medical courses at home. Within the government, new plans were being discussed for a medical facility that would educate women. Again, however, they were waylaid by the flinty opposition of Tolstoy, now Minister of the Interior. Not until Tolstoy left the government in the early 1890s could the concept move forward. When it became known that finances were a major stumbling block, a new wave of donations came from people and organizations throughout the Empire. Medical organizations meanwhile kept up their demands that women be allowed to study medicine.[65] A petition from a large convention of Russian doctors in 1892 was drawn up by Friedrich Erismann, the Swiss-born champion of public health in Russia. Citing the huge lack of doctors in the Empire, he praised the performance of women in bringing health care to thousands in need and urged that their number be increased.[66]

## Triumph and Chaos

The crucial decisions were made in 1894–95. Concern over the perils of foreign study figured importantly in the final outcome. In 1894 the head of the secret police warned the government that nearly half of the women medical students in Switzerland and Paris were disloyal to their country. Graduates of the courses in St. Petersburg, on the other hand, had far better records. It was his recommendation that women be trained once more in Russia to "protect them from the pernicious influence of the emigrés and facilitate the development in them of a political attitude more favorable to the government."[67] On the first day of June, 1895, the project to found a medical institute for women was approved by the new Tsar, Nicholas II.

The final years of Imperial Russia were marked by a burst of medical study by women unknown in any other country. The new Women's Medical Institute, built to handle fifteen hundred students, was opened in St. Petersburg in 1897. It became the favorite charity of groups and individuals all across Russia. Scholarships were founded; new institutes and clinics were added to the original buildings; and professors gave freely of their time and money to make the Institute a success. The curriculum was fully equal to that of the other medical schools in Russia, and the government gave recognition to its graduates as equal with men in medical practice. Most of the funds to run the Institute now came from the government. Restrictions on the personal and political behavior of students, however, were as tight as in the previous women's medical courses. A further disturbing note was the virtual exclusion of Jewish women, who had made up 20 percent of the final classes in the previous courses. The laws of 1886 had limited Jewish students to 3 percent of the student body in cities such as St. Petersburg, and this quota was now applied to the Institute.[68]

Women flocked to the new courses. By 1903, enrollment had reached nearly fourteen hundred students. At its peak in 1906, 1,635 women were studying medicine in St. Petersburg. Another four to five hundred applicants were being turned away each year. Students came from as far away as eastern Siberia, the northern provinces, the Caspian Sea, and the Caucasus. About 20 percent were supported by scholarships from *zemstvos,* cities, and private benefactors. The facilities were the best provided for women in Russia and were superior to those of the women's schools in Great Britain and America. Provision was made for an impressive range of faculty positions, all held by male professors. An atmosphere of learning and research, it was reported by Western visitors, prevailed in the Institute; faculty

members and instructors (*dotsenty*) were expected to make original
investigations and, so far as possible, to involve the students.[69]

Some of those refused admission turned to the new medical
schools for women in Moscow (1907), Kiev (1907), Odessa (1909),
or Kharkov (1910). Additional schools were built before the collapse
of the Tsarist government in 1917. Enrollment at Kiev alone reached
1,224 in 1913, while the school in Kharkov counted 1,558 women
the same year. Over half of the student bodies of these two schools
came from lower-middle-class or peasant families, as these were
defined by law. Jewish women, severely restricted in Moscow and
St. Petersburg, were sometimes able to gain admission to the provincial programs for women. In Odessa, for example, despite a quota,
the proportion of Jewish women in the medical courses reached 12
percent. When the quota was dropped altogether during the war,
they quickly took over half of the places in the medical program.[70]

The revolutionary conditions after 1900 created chaos in the medical schools. Students were affected by the continuing upheavals as
the government alternately closed and reopened the schools. The
Women's Medical Institute had closed twice by the spring of 1905
and many students had been arrested. Jews, Poles, and other non-
Russian women, as well as those seeking asylum, left Russia in droves
to take up study in Switzerland or France. After the Revolution of
1905, which led to the temporary closing of all institutions of higher
learning, as many as fifteen hundred Russian women were studying
medicine abroad. At home, the government sought to placate students in the aftermath of 1905. Women's courses were expanded;
women were again allowed as auditors in the universities; and the
universities were given autonomy over their own affairs. The total
number of women students in Russia (all fields) jumped swiftly from
six thousand in 1904 to forty-four thousand in 1915, or a third of
all students in the Empire.[71]

The campus of the Women's Medical Institute was rocked by
strikes and demonstrations in the years after 1910. In the spring of
1914, education came to a complete standstill as students went on
strike in support of industrial workers in the city. The outbreak of
war brought a period of patriotic closing of ranks; many students
volunteered to help in caring for the wounded. In March 1917,
however, the women took part in the final riots that ended the Tsar's
rule. A year later, the Institute was thrown open to all applicants by

the Bolsheviks and nearly fifteen hundred new students, men and women, were allowed to enter.[72]

By the time of the Tsar's fall, the number of women practicing medicine in Russia had reached five thousand.[73] Thousands more were still in medical school, and still others were seeking state approval of degrees taken abroad. Everywhere there was a sense of women in motion, of seismic changes in women's historic position. Well before the Soviet takeover, Russian women had achieved a level of participation in medicine unrivaled in any other country. They had overcome fierce resistance from governmental authorities and obstacles that are only now beginning to be understood. At least seven or eight thousand of them had taken long journeys abroad, where loneliness, a strange language, and lack of money often brought further misery. Many who went abroad were Jewish women who sought to escape the harsh legal and social discriminations imposed on them in Russia. At home, all of the women faced the agonizing wait for a place to study, the capricious quotas on their enrollment, and the many bars to full professional participation after graduation. Those who won a chance at practice had already proven themselves in the eyes of the public and much of officialdom. As Erismann described it, they had long since demonstrated the physical strength to handle the long hours, the country visits, and the great distances traveled over bad roads in rural Russia. They had performed, he said, the most delicate operations in general surgery, gynecology, and ophthalmology. "Women doctors in Russia," he told his Swiss and German countrymen, "are sometimes preferred" in the city as well as in the country.[74]

The Russian example had a powerful effect on women's struggle for education throughout Europe. Without question, the success of so many Russian women in medicine in the West gave encouragement to native women. When they returned to Russia, they gave new force to the arguments for coeducation in medicine and other fields at home. Western visitors to the women's medical schools in Russia after 1897 consistently praised the teaching and facilities for women. "Russian women's medical education," writes one historian, "had no equal in Europe in facilities, faculty, and curriculum."[75]

One nation that was influenced by the Russian example was Imperial Germany. Longer than any other Western nation, Germany kept women out of its universities and discouraged efforts to build separate schools for them. When the argument over admitting women to medicine was raging at the end of the nineteenth century, both German defenders of women's study and their opponents pointed to the example of the Russian women or cited experiences they had had with Russian women students in Swiss universities. A score of books and articles were published in Germany and Austria that looked to the question of women physicians in light of the Russian achievement.[76] A typical article pointed to the deep respect in which Russian women physicians were held by their countrymen and the stamina with which they took their skills to all parts of Russia.[77] The fight to bring German women into the medical schools, to which we now turn, owed much to what had happened in Zurich, Paris, and St. Petersburg.

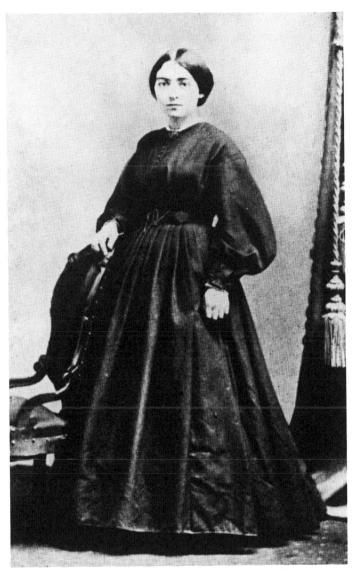

Mary Corinna Putnam, pioneer American medical woman abroad, in 1866

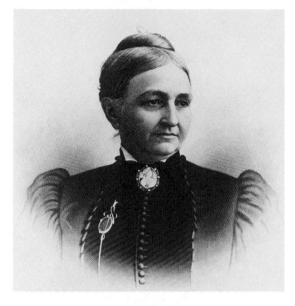

Mary H. Thompson, founder of Chicago's medical
college for women

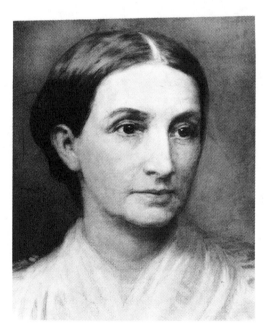

Ann Preston, graduate and early dean of the
Woman's Medical College of Pennsylvania

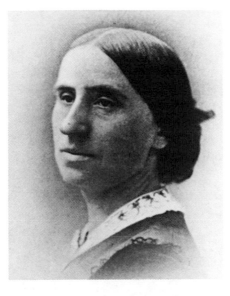

Marie Zakrzewska, leader of the women's
medical profession in Boston, about 1870

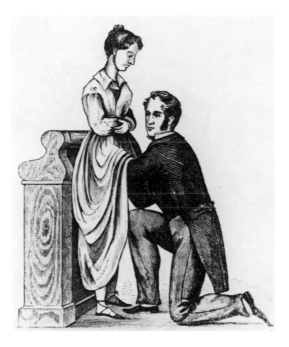

An obstetrical examination as pictured in Samuel
Gregory's *Medical Morals* (ca. 1852)

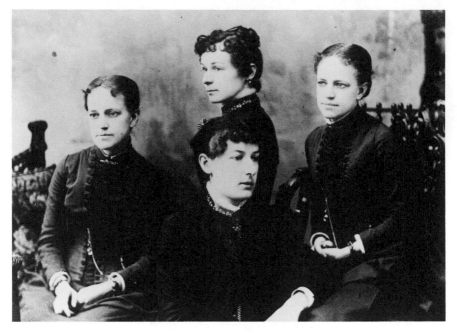

Four American women who studied medicine in Paris: Emily Pope, C. Augusta Pope, Agnes Lowry, Isabel Lowry

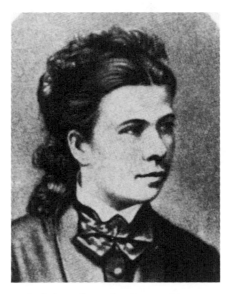

Nadezhda Suslova, the first modern woman to earn a medical degree in a recognized university

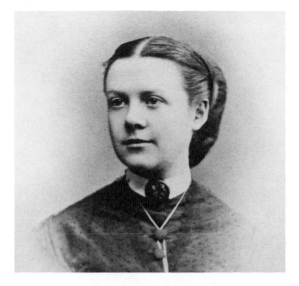

Susan Dimock, early American woman surgeon and
graduate of Zurich

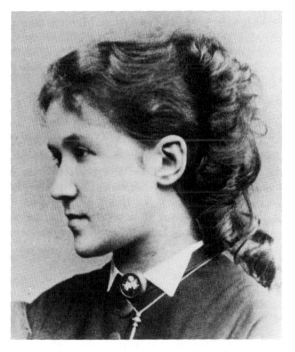

Maria Bokova, a heroine to a generation of Russian
women

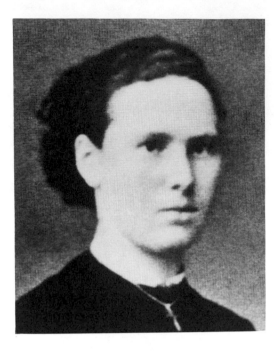

Elizabeth Morgan, who created a legend in Zurich

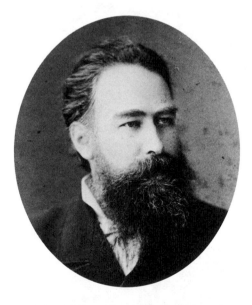

Friedrich Erismann, Swiss physician who
married Nadezhda Suslova and became a
high public health official in Russia

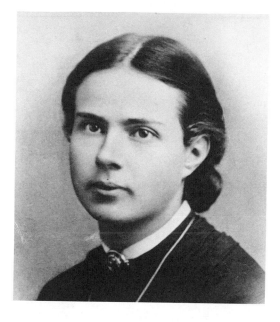

Marie Vögtlin, the first Swiss woman to graduate
in medicine

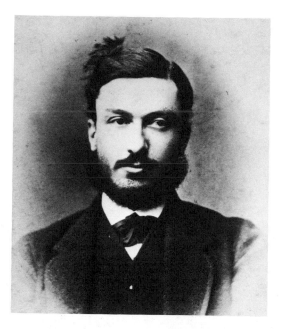

August Forel, psychiatrist and classmate
of Nadezhda Suslova at Zurich

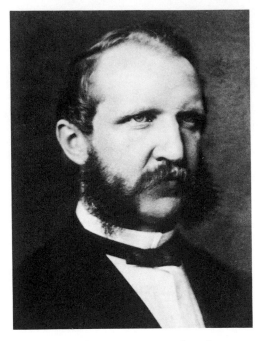

Edmund Rose, Swiss surgeon and professor
who supported women's medical education

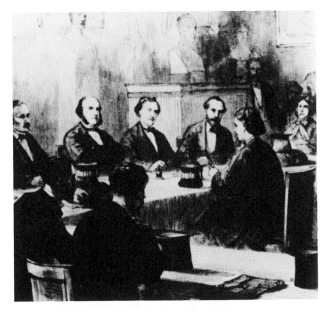

Elizabeth Garrett taking her oral examination in Paris

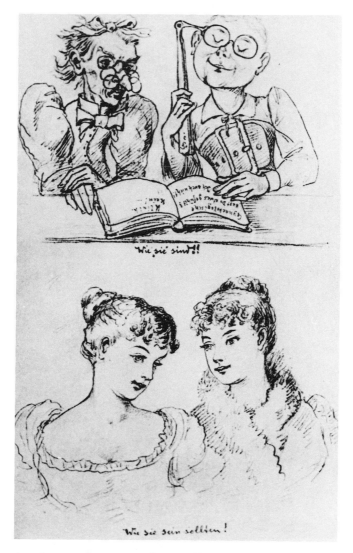

A caricature of women students in Zurich. Above: "How they are!" Below: "How they should be!"

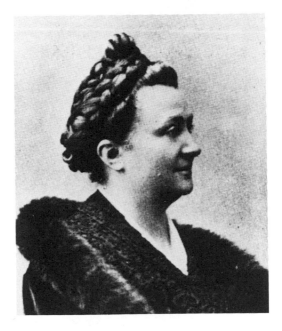

Madeleine Brès, leader of the women's medical profession in Paris

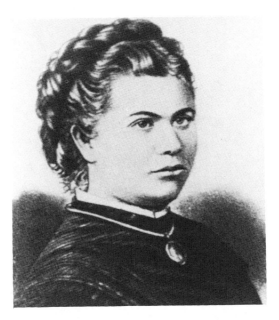

Varvara Kashevarova, the first woman to complete her medical studies in Russia

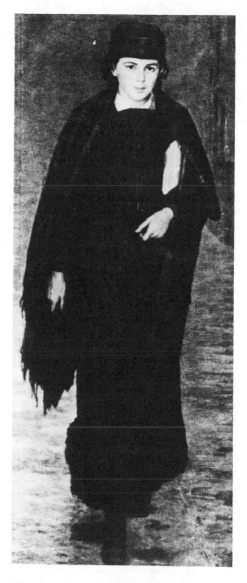

A Russian woman student of the early
1880s, from a painting by Nikolaj Jarošenko

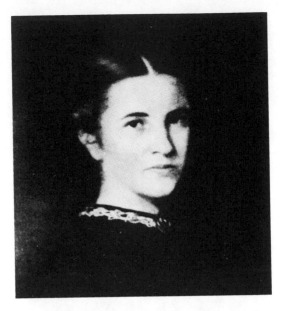

Elizabeth Garrett Anderson as dean of the London
School of Medicine for Women

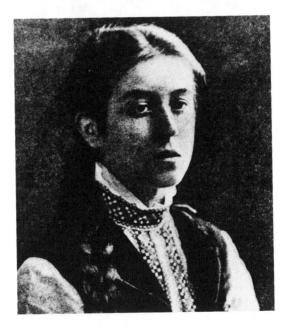

Vera Figner, a Zurich medical student who was
later sentenced to death in the assassination of
Czar Alexander II

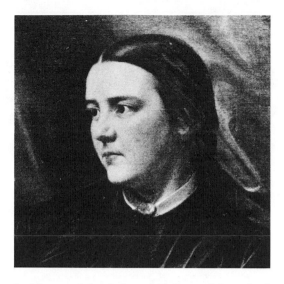

Sophia Jex-Blake, firebrand of the English medical
women's movement

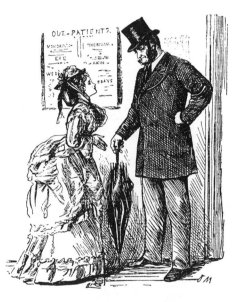

Cartoon on "The Coming Race" from *Punch*. Captions read:
Doctor Evangeline: "Mr. Sawyer, are you engaged
tomorrow afternoon? I have rather a ticklish operation."
Mr. Sawyer: "I shall be happy to do it for you."
Doctor Evangeline: "O, no, not that! But will you
kindly come and administer the chloroform for me?"

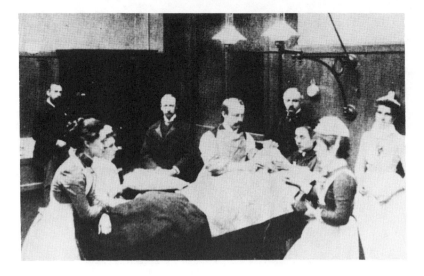

Clinical instruction at the London School of Medicine for Women in the late nineteenth century

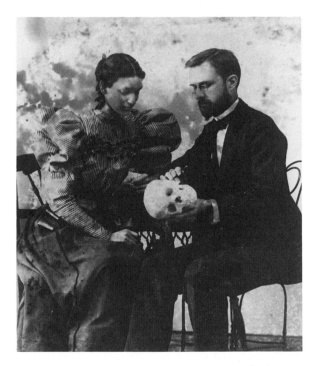

A student and her teacher at the Woman's Medical College of Pennsylvania, ca. 1895

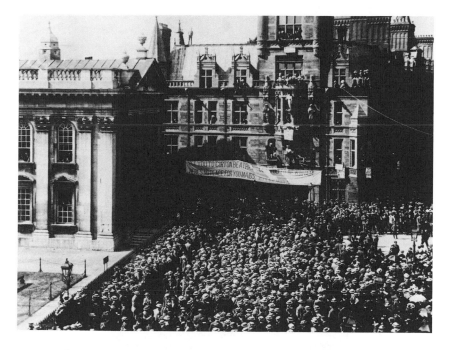

Cambridge University students protesting the admission of women, 1897

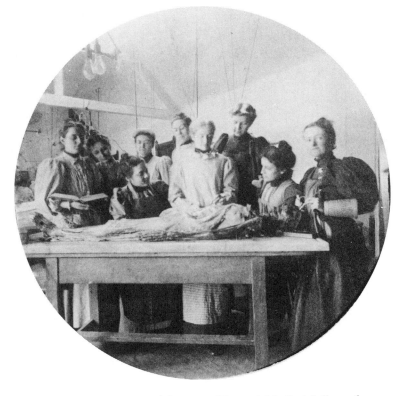

Students in anatomy laboratory, Woman's Medical College of
Pennsylvania, class of 1897

# 5  *Imperial Germany*

To the women of Germany, the achievement of Russia's medical women must have seemed spectacular indeed. Until 1900, no woman had been fully trained in medicine anywhere in Germany. As late as 1913, when Russian women accounted for 10 percent of the profession in that country, there were only 138 women physicians in the entire German Reich.[1] Medical enrollment of women did not reach one thousand students until the summer of 1914, when the comparable figure in Russia was four times that number (Table 5).[2] During the preceding half-century, Russia had been constantly far ahead of Germany in the number of its women who sought higher education both at home and abroad.

Curiously, though, the Russian example was used by German opponents as proof of the great danger in allowing women to study medicine. The radical, unconventional lifestyles of the Russian

*Table 5.*   German and Russian women matriculated in medical school, 1880–1914

|            | 1880 | 1900 | 1914  |
|------------|------|------|-------|
| Russia     | 504  | 920  | 4,414 |
| Germany    | 0    | 8    | 1,027 |

*Sources:* The Russian figures are based on the number of women admitted to the women's medical courses and the data in Ruth Dudgeon, "A Forgotten Minority: Women Students in Imperial Russia, 1872–1917," *Russian History/Histoire Russe,* 1982, 9: 9–20. The German figures are taken from Elisabeth Burger, "Die Entwicklung des medizinischen Frauenstudiums" (doctoral dissertation, University of Marburg, 1947), p. 53, and exclude student auditors.

women in Zurich were seen by German critics as confirmation of their deep fears of university study by women. The Russian *ukase* of 1873, which was widely reported in Germany, had been explicit in its accusations of sexual immorality among the medical women. It even charged them with studying obstetrics abroad in order to perform illegal abortions at home. A Tübingen gynecologist spoke for many when he cited the "dubious moral behavior" of the Russian women as grounds for excluding them from his university.[3] Fears were also expressed that German women might become radicalized through university study or adopt the strange habits and dress of the Russian women. A careful modern historian has described the Zurich experience as "extremely detrimental to the nascent movement for female physicians in Germany."[4]

But the roots of German backwardness in educating women lay deeper in German history and culture. "What was unique to Germany," writes Gordon Craig, "was that the subordination of women was more stubborn and protracted than in the advanced Western countries."[5] In the period of reaction that followed the revolutions of 1848, earlier cries for women's rights and a chance at education were largely stilled in the German states. Marie Zakrzewska, growing up in Berlin in these years, found the atmosphere of puritanical repression and male authoritarianism suffocating to women. "Each [German] man," she wrote, "thinks himself the lord of creation and, of course, regards woman only as his appendage."[6]

Women were everywhere tightly bound by legal restrictions and social conventions that went far beyond those of Britain and America. No strong liberal movement took up their cause as in Britain or France. Churches and other conservative organizations reinforced their subordination. The continuing political division of Germany made a free association of women reformers across state lines at best problematical. While more and more women were being forced to enter the labor force in the last half of the century, the barriers to careers in government and the professions remained insurmountable. "What is the reason the German woman can not obtain what the women of other civilized nations obtained?" demanded Helene Lange in 1890. "Is the reason to be looked for in themselves? Or in the men? Or in insurmountable exterior obstacles?"[7]

For Lange, the answer lay in the women themselves and only partly in external conditions and the hostile attitude of German men.

Germany lacked a strong women's movement comparable to that of Britain or America. The German *Hausfrau,* she argued, was too smugly preoccupied with her own interests and those of her family. She showed no concern for her unmarried sisters and those now forced by necessity to look for employment. She was too much the captive of deeply rooted beliefs about woman's proper role in the family. She failed to enlist the support of husbands and brothers in the fight to tear down the barriers faced by women who needed to work. The German women's movement was therefore not well supported and was frequently divided and ineffective.[8]

More sharply than in other countries, the women's movement in Germany was split into separate movements of middle-class and working-class women. The growing socialist movement claimed the allegiance of many working women. For those in the middle class, the chance for an education, political and legal rights, and the ending of job discrimination were overarching goals, while women employed in industry tended to focus on the conditions of work in the factories, trade-union action, and socialistic goals for the larger society.[9] This division of forces, in the face of the granitic opposition to change in women's position in Wilhelmine Germany, clearly made the task of educational reform more difficult.

In neighboring Austria, the prospects for women's study were scarcely better. The Austrian women's movement, though less divided, was weak and faced equally determined opposition. Women's opportunities for secondary education were long restricted, as in Germany, to private and church schools and to a few public schools. The universities of Austria were tightly closed to them until the end of the century. As late as 1912, no woman had been trained in law or theology in any university in Austria.[10]

In both Germany and Austria, the fight for women's higher education was protracted and bitter. As in Russia, the first study by women began outside the formal structure of the universities. It was supported by such women's organizations as the Lette-Verein and the Allgemeine Deutsche Frauenverein, both founded in 1865. The purpose of the Lette-Verein, according to one of its leaders, was "to discover new occupations fitted for women, to protect their interests in those where they already have a footing, and to educate them for more important and profitable employments."[11] The Allgemeine Deutsche Frauenverein, on the other hand, stressed the creation of lyceums or secondary schools and "advanced scientific training" for women. The lyceum courses for young women, like the early higher education courses in Russia, were informal and loosely structured. They were described by the American educator Hugh Puckett as a "somewhat desultory feeding of the young ladies' minds with lectures of university grade, without expecting them to make more than a cultural use of it."[12] Not until Helene Lange founded her "Realkurse" in Berlin in 1889 was there a German school specifically aimed at preparing women for university study.[13]

The conservative political order affected deeply the professors who guided the universities. They were, in effect, officials of the state and seldom challenged the fundamental principles and values of German society. Those who sympathized with the liberal currents of reform of 1830 and 1848, as we have seen, frequently found refuge in Zurich and Bern. Unlike Russia, America, France, or Britain, few voices were raised in German medical schools in favor of allowing women a chance at professional education. Even those who had shared in the experience in educating women at Zurich usually maintained a strict silence when they later won a chair at a German university. As a result, the medical world of Germany maintained its solid front against women more successfully than any other nation.

For a brief period in the 1860s and 1870s, before attitudes began to harden, it seemed that Germany might follow the Russian lead in admitting women informally to the universities. The University of Munich, as early as 1865, had declared its readiness to admit women to medical lectures. At least sixteen women attended various courses in the medical school before the authorities, in the face of growing criticism, decided to discontinue the practice.[14] The faculty senate of the University of Königsberg asked the Prussian Ministry of Culture in 1871 for permission to admit women to the medical school, but the request was denied.[15] In Leipzig, according to university records, a small number of women were allowed to audit university courses, including medicine, between 1873 and 1882. The American educator M. Carey Thomas wrote from Germany of the "conflicting accounts" about Leipzig's being open to women, probably because of the differing policies followed by individual schools and faculty members.[16] Another American woman reported in 1879 that there were eight women at the University, including one in medicine.[17] Heidelberg, too, allowed a few women auditors to attend lectures. Here and there, a woman was allowed to take a degree. Leipzig, for example, awarded a law degree to a Russian woman of German heritage in 1873.[18] The following year, the brilliant Russian mathematician Sofia Kovalevskaia was allowed to take a doctorate in Göttingen. Further research in university archives would doubtless produce other examples of such exceptional actions. From what is known at this time, however, such cases were limited to a few women in a handful of universities.

## Verboten: The Ban on Women in Medicine

The sudden crisis of the early 1870s in Zurich, which was the only German-language university fully open to women, brought the first serious attention to the issue of women's study to Germany. A number of the Russian women banned from further study in Zurich turned to German universities in their frantic efforts to find a new place to study. In Göttingen, a request from a Russian woman to be admitted to study medicine was rejected by the medical faculty.[19] Others were denied admission at Leipzig, Freiburg, Tübingen, Strassburg, Giessen, Erlangen, and Rostock. When two Russian women petitioned the University of Heidelberg to allow them to attend medical lectures in the summer of 1873 the faculty senate passed a resolution forbidding women "totally" with the "exception of those ladies who have already begun their studies."[20]

At Munich, in 1872, Theodor von Bischoff published his savage attack on the Zurich experiment in educating Russian and other women in medicine. Bischoff was the most influential anatomist in Germany, and his pamphlet was widely discussed and quoted. The arguments he used—the lack of physical stamina in women, their lesser brain capacity, their emotional nature, their effect on male students—were repeated scores of times over the next three decades. "One thing is certain," he concluded in Darwinian fashion, "the strongest always wins and proves himself thereby the stronger." This was demonstrated "in the victory of men everywhere in all circumstances in science and the [medical] profession." His own position at Munich was completely clear: "I personally . . . am unshakably determined never to permit women in my lectures."[21]

Among the women in Zurich when Bischoff levied his attack were two medical students from Germany. Emilie Lehmus, the daughter of a Bavarian pastor in Fürth, was twenty-nine years old when she arrived in Zurich in the fall of 1870. Her German friend Franziska Tiburtius, who came the following year, described her as a woman of "delicate build, with lively, dark eyes, glowing countenance, and quick, very agile movements."[22] Extremely bright, Lehmus graduated *summa cum laude* after nine semesters. Tiburtius, whose family lived on the island of Rügen in the forbidding Baltic Sea, had been a teacher for six years and had been preparing to open a girls' school before her brother convinced her to study medicine. Both she and Lehmus were inspired by the example of her sister-in-law, Henriette Tiburtius-Hirschfeld, who had crossed the Atlantic to study dentistry in the United States and then started a successful practice in Berlin.[23] For Tiburtius, the decision to leave home and family for Zurich was agonizing. "A young girl at a university and studying medicine— unthinkable!" she later wrote.[24] At Zurich she did well in her studies and graduated in 1876. Her fellow students found her serious, hard-working, and very reserved. A Russian woman commented that she was "somewhat stiff" and "thoroughly correct," someone to "respect rather than a fellow student."[25] After graduation both women sought clinical experience in Germany, but only the gynecologist Franz von Winckel at Dresden was willing to take them into his clinic as voluntary physicians. For the next quarter-century, Winckel would be one of the very few German professors to welcome women to postgraduate opportunities in medicine.

The efforts of Tiburtius and Lehmus to gain employment after graduation did not encourage other German women to take up medical study. They were not allowed to apply for a medical license or even to take the examinations in midwifery. After two years in Berlin, the women opened a modest polyclinic for women with the sufferance of Prussian authorities. It was "heavy, uphill work" to establish a small practice among the poorer women of the city.[26] Support came chiefly from family, friends, and patients. A friendly Berlin industrialist, for example, gave them a house suitable for use as a clinic. The city's physicians ignored them or treated them with contempt. When Tiburtius and Lehmus were about to deliver a lecture one day at the Victoria Lyceum in the city, the pathologist Rudolf Virchow ostentatiously walked out of the auditorium.[27]

For the next dozen years, the two Zurich graduates were the only women physicians in Berlin. More women left for Zurich, but few completed their studies to return to a hostile environment at home. Some of the women were helped by scholarships from women's groups in Germany.[28] In all, fourteen additional German women, including Anna Kuhnow, Agnes Bluhm, Agnes Hacker, and Pauline Plötz, all of whom settled in Berlin, completed their M.D. degrees in Zurich in the years before 1900.[29] Another ninety-one women left Germany to study medicine in Zurich before the end of the century, but the records do not tell us what happened to such women as Josepha Haag of Strassburg, Dora Schimper of Zweibrücken, Mathilde Heumann of Darmstadt, or Dorothea Hahn of Hamburg.[30]

A smaller number of Austrian women left their homeland to study in Switzerland. Only four of them had taken their medical degrees by the end of the century. Of these, Sarah Welt left Austria to practice in New York, while her sister, Leonore, remained in Switzerland after her graduation.[31] Only Gabriele von Possaner, a baroness from Vienna, who studied in Zurich from 1889 to 1894, made active efforts to practice in Austria. Her Swiss degree was at first given no recognition, and appeals to officials and state courts were uniformly turned down. Only a petition to the emperor finally brought results, but even then, she was required to repeat all of her examinations at the University of Vienna before being admitted to practice in May 1897.[32] In the meantime, several other women had been given special permission to practice in Austria, and some Swiss-trained women were sent to treat Moslem women in Bosnia.[33]

For thirty years, following the departure of Emilie Lehmus for Zurich, the ban on women's study in Imperial Germany and Austria was the most stringent of the advanced industrial countries. Emigration was the only way for women to gain any training at all in medicine. Private medical colleges for women of the sort that began in the United States and that later sprang up in Russia and Britain were useless in a state where universities had the exclusive right to prepare physicians for the medical profession. Women were additionally banned from the humanistic gymnasia, which alone prepared students for the university.

The success of foreign women in becoming doctors was dismissed by German authorities as irrelevant to German conditions. German savants debated the issue almost entirely from the viewpoint of their own attitudes and experience, disregarded or ignored conflicting evidence, and refused to take seriously reports of women's success in the United States, Zurich, Paris, or Russia. "The example of Russia," wrote Dr. Leopold Henius in the *Deutsche medicinische Wochenschrift,* "cannot be considered worthy of emulation," for the Russians had simply made a virtue out of necessity in trying to provide physicians for the vast stretches of Russian territory that were not served by doctors.[34] Max Runge of Göttingen, agreeing, said that in Russia and America "female doctors are [probably] better than no doctors at all."[35] Even Frances Morgan, the redoubtable Englishwoman at Zurich, who had become a member of the Association of German Naturalists and Physicians, did not escape censure. She was abruptly removed from the Association's rolls in 1879 after a speaker urged his colleagues to purge themselves "of the presence of women."[36] Victor Böhmert, who had seen women's medical education at first hand in Zurich, chided his German colleagues for continually condemning women's study "without having had any experience" with it.[37]

## The Bitter Debate

The vehemence of the opposition of German professors and physicians to women's study exceeded that of any other country. No quarter was asked or given in the fight to protect Germany from the "foreign custom" of allowing women to study side by side with men.[38] "I wish I could convey to thee," Carey Thomas wrote her mother, "an idea of the way women are mentioned by the profs and in German books."[39] All of the arguments heard in other countries for denying women a chance at medicine were clothed in Wilhelmine Germany with a heavy coat of sarcasm, labored logic, and scientific veneer. The biological argument of women's physical inferiority, for example, was carried much further in Germany than elsewhere. In addition to Bischoff's precise anatomical data on the size and weight of the female skull and brain, other scientists such as the neurologist Paul Möbius, the Viennese surgeon E. Albert, and the Berlin physician Leopold Henius wrote at length of the disabling physical constitution of the weaker sex. In his provocatively titled treatise "On the Physiological Inferiority [*Schwachsinn*] of the Female," which went through eight editions, Möbius cited a number of studies to prove that the parts of the brain that were critical for mental performance were far less developed in women than in men.⁴⁰ Albert, on the other hand, was convinced that women could never physically stand up to the "long, nightly marches" to distant patients. Imagine, he said, a doctor called from sleep to tramp three hours in the snow-covered Alps to attend a difficult case of childbirth "that demands the greatest mental and physical exertions . . . Would you wish such an existence for your gifted daughter?"⁴¹ For Henius, the weak musculature and bone structure of women made medical study and active practice a positive danger to their health. "If we look at the younger ladies from the circles that [are pushing] the study of medicine," he wrote, "we find no strong, blooming sex, on the contrary, the young girls of today are for the most part, despite careful nurture, anemic, miserable, and frail."⁴²

The gynecologists of the Reich added fuel to the controversy by continuing to stress menstruation as a particularly incapacitating weakness of women. According to Professor Hermann Fehling, all of the physiological measurements of women—pulse, blood pressure, body temperature, muscle strength, lung capacity—showed that bodily function reached its peak just before menstruation. At the middle point between menstrual periods, conversely, all of these measurements were at their lowest point. These scientific observations, he said, pointed to a constant waxing and waning of not only the physical but also the mental functions of the woman.⁴³ This physical changeability was characterized by his colleague Max Runge as "a condition of irritable weakness" that made the woman doctor undependable at critical moments.⁴⁴

The German attack on women's suitability for medicine put heavy stress, too, on their delicate "psyche," which unsuited them for the bloody realities of medical practice. Women were too sensitive, too emotional, too inexperienced, to manage the life-and-death decisions made every day by physicians and surgeons. "There is nothing more unfeminine," said Professor Franz Riegel of Göttingen, "than the surgical knife."⁴⁵ Women, said Fehling, had difficulty in distinguishing what was essential from the inessential in decisionmaking at the bedside.⁴⁶ For many critics, it was simply not possible to reconcile the traditional picture of a woman with the demanding intellectual and physical qualities needed by a physician. "Independent thought, logic, thirst for knowledge, capacity for abstraction, reverence for ideas and principles, the search for connections and the whole, and

the inventive spirit," writes Raymond Hollmann, "represented together the advantage of the masculine mind which, if they were
strongly impregnated in a woman, would mean the loss of 'genuine'
femininity."[47] Almost no German writer believed that woman's central role of housewife and mother could be combined with the practice of a profession.

A few German physicians did take up their pens to defend the
capacities of women. Almost all of them had experienced women's
study abroad. Ludimar Hermann, for example, who had defended
the Zurich experiment against Bischoff's assault in 1872, continued
to take a moderate stand on the issue after his appointment in Königsberg.[48] The gynecologist Adolf Gusserow and the pathologist
Georg Rindfleisch, both of whom had spent time in Zurich, commented that "during the entire time of [our] observation [in Zurich]
there was never any inconvenience from the common study of men
and women students."[49] From Moscow the respected public health
expert Friedrich Erismann, a former student at Zurich, reported in
the pages of a German women's magazine on the remarkable achievements of Russian women doctors.[50] In New York, the German-
American pediatrician Abraham Jacobi told German physicians in
1896 that "many years ago" there had been the same kind of resistance to women doctors in America as was now reported in the
German press. But today, he reported, "it is no more unusual to see
a woman come to a medical society [meeting] and sit right in front
as to see one on a street car." None of the terrible consequences
predicted for women's study had come to pass. Coeducation, he
advised, was superior to separate schools for women. "It will not be
long," he concluded, "before you have women doctors" and German
medical classes will have "less noise, fewer duels, more decorum,
and more work."[51]

The gynecologist Franz von Winckel, who had given so many
women advanced training in his clinics at Dresden and Munich,
spoke favorably of his twenty years of working with women. "I have
had to recognize with pleasure the achievements of most of these
women as at least equal to those of their fellow voluntary physicians," he wrote in 1897. "Even the most delicate among them were
able to carry out difficult operations successfully."[52] More than forty
women, some of them foreign, many trained in Zurich, had come
to him to get clinical experience in women's diseases.[53] "I find it

very noteworthy and very good-hearted of Professor Winckel," Tiburtius wrote her brother from Dresden, "that he is swimming
against the current and accepts us here . . . [It] is the only place in
Germany . . . to get experience, and we must be thankful for it."[54]
It is not clear why Winckel, alone among the outstanding medical
men of Germany, should have taken so progressive a position for so
long in regard to women's education.


## The Turn of the Tide

By the time of Winckel's public praise for women doctors in 1897,
the tide of medical and public opinion had clearly begun to turn.
The first signs of change can be traced to the late 1880s, when the
women's movement entered a new phase. Helene Lange had written
an influential pamphlet in 1887 that sharply attacked the idea that
women should be educated only to suit the needs of their husbands.
She demanded a complete reform in women's education, with
women themselves playing an important role in their own instruction.[55] A flurry of petitions, often accompanied by the pamphlet, was
sent by the Allgemeine Deutsche Frauenverein to the education min-
istries of the German states as well as to the Reichstag asking that
the universities and professions be opened to women. New and more
radical women's groups joined in the struggle to win professional
training for women. A new energy and hopefulness were apparent
in the ranks of their leaders. The retirement of Bismarck and the
lapsing of the antisocialist laws in 1890 encouraged a more open
political atmosphere.[56] Census studies that same year revealed that
the Reich now contained a million more women than men and that
2.2 million women were widows. It was clear that not all German
women would be able to fulfill their "natural calling" as housewives
and mothers. As a contemporary writer phrased it, "they cannot
marry, yet still want to exist."[57]

The new campaign was sharply focused on opening medical study
to women. This strategy was rooted in the belief that opposition was
weakening to the idea of women being treated by doctors of their
own sex. An important weapon in this strategy was a small book
written by Mathilde Weber in 1888 entitled *Female Physicians for
Women's Diseases: An Ethical and Sanitary Necessity.* Weber, the wife

of a Tübingen professor, insisted that women physicians must be educated in Germany so that thousands of women who avoided seeing a doctor out of feelings of shame or delicacy could be protected in their modesty. Women doctors were badly needed, too, in girls' schools and women's prisons.[58] The book became instantly a subject of wide discussion in governmental and academic circles.

Weber then carried her campaign to Zurich, where, she reported, she found none of the crude behavior among women students reported in the German press. "Where then [is] the extravagant, unfeminine behavior feared by such opponents as Herr Professor Dr. Bischoff," she asked, "where [are] the oft-pictured cigarettes and men's clothing?" She found among the German women, she said, "only fresh, strong women, mostly widows, and girls full of womanly decency." The widespread prejudice against women medical students in Zurich, she insisted, went back to the early Russians who had differing "social views" and "cultural background" than West Europeans. The women she saw were serious about their studies, well behaved, appropriately dressed, and led a "truly cloistered life." She praised especially the Swiss men who were "the first in Europe to provide an example of objective fairness for our sex." Thus did she hope to persuade her own countrymen to provide a similar chance for women in Germany.[59]

The political struggle over women doctors seesawed back and forth between the various state governments and the federal parliament. Some states and universities were more sympathetic than others to the idea of educating women in medicine. The individual states, furthermore, had retained a large measure of autonomy in educational matters in the Second Reich, yet the national government was clearly interested, too, in a social question so politically significant as the legal rights of women. The licensure of physicians, moreover, was administered in Berlin and not in the states. When the Reichstag turned down their first petition in 1890 to open medical licensure to women, the women's groups prepared a new request, this time with 55,000 signatures.[60] Step by step, the federal and state governments moved closer each year to lowering the bars to women in medicine. In 1892, the House of Deputies in Prussia expressed itself in favor of opening medical schools to women. A survey of the Prussian universities at the same time showed four of the nine medical faculties in favor of the idea. The Prussian Minister of Education moved in 1895 to allow women to take the *Abitur* (high school diploma), which would make them eligible for university study. Only the threat of Ernst von Bergmann, the doyen of German surgeons, to resign from the University of Berlin stopped him from opening the medical schools of Prussia immediately to women. In 1897, the school of medicine at Freiburg in Baden resolved to seek approval to matriculate women. Abroad, Austria opened its universities to women in 1897 and its medical faculties in 1900, while Russia had begun its new medical school for women in St. Petersburg. All these events were widely reported in Germany. Finally, in 1899, the federal Bundesrat, succumbing to the pressure, approved the granting of medical licenses to women.[61]

The struggle was not yet over. It remained for the individual states to open their medical schools to women. Throughout the latter 1880s and the 1890s a number of them began once more to permit women to attend university lectures as auditors. Normally, special permission from the professor and sometimes from the university and state authorities was required to attend a particular course. As auditors, the women could not count on having these courses recognized as normal medical study toward examinations or a degree. These "hearers" were exposed, of course, to the curiosity of other students and sometimes to rudeness at the hands of a professor. Permission to hear the lectures could be withdrawn at any time. In Munich, according to the historian Johannes Steudel, the mere presence of a woman at one controversial medical lecture caused permission to attend classes to be withdrawn from all women auditors.[62]

Among the first women allowed to attend lectures in these years were a number of Americans eager to study in a German university. At the University of Leipzig, for example, women from the United States were prominent among those auditing classes in several subjects between 1886 and 1893.[63] Göttingen, too, opened its doors unofficially to a small group of women in 1893. Three women, two of them American, were admitted to lectures in the school of philosophy (that is, liberal arts) in Göttingen that fall. Two years later, the first medical auditor, also an American, joined a group of thirty-two women at the University. The medical student, Florence Dyer of Boston, who had attended the Woman's Medical College of Pennsylvania, was sponsored inadvertently by the pathologist Johannes Orth, who mistook her application for that of a man. In all, thirty-seven women studied medicine at Göttingen before women were officially allowed to matriculate in 1908.[64]

Other universities followed in permitting women to audit particular classes. The University of Berlin, which welcomed its first woman in 1895, became very popular among both German and foreign women. By 1908, the number of women attending classes unofficially in Berlin reached 508, of whom 82 were studying medicine.[65] Freiburg was likewise popular, especially with foreign students. After turning down an American woman who wanted to study medicine in 1890, the university reversed itself and awarded a doctoral degree in zoology to an American, Elizabeth Bickford, in 1895, as well as a medical degree to a Dutch woman the same year.[66] Other foreign women, especially Russians, began to appear at Freiburg and other places in the middle 1890s. By the summer of 1901, 22 of the 24 women auditing courses in medicine at Leipzig were foreigners.[67] The universities that barred women completely were becoming a minority. Only six of the twenty universities in the Reich, according to a survey in 1896, were still closed entirely to women.[68] More than a thousand women were attending lectures in German universities by the early twentieth century, including 95 in medicine.[69]

This idiosyncratic pattern of allowing women into universities created a number of contradictions. Women barred from attending lectures in a university at home might be welcomed at another university fifty miles away. A woman listening to lectures in history or medieval German might be refused attendance in a course in anatomy. A medical student could be allowed to attend lectures in physiology but not in anatomy. Ilse Szagunn of Berlin, for example, had to take a private course in anatomy because the famous Wilhelm Waldeyer of the Berlin faculty allowed no women in his anatomy course.[70] The countess Maria von Linden, who was granted a doctorate *cum laude* in the science school at Tübingen, was forced to go to Zurich to take medical courses because Tübingen's medical faculty would not admit her.[71] At Heidelberg, an American woman, Ida Hyde, was awarded a doctorate in physiology in 1896 after the University of Strassburg, where she had been studying, refused to give her a degree. Even then, Willy Kühne, the renowned physiologist, balked at serving on her committee and refused to concur in the *summa cum laude* recommendation of his colleagues.[72]

The growing pressure to grant women full admission caused some to advocate the "American Solution" of separate medical schools. Others argued for at least separate classes for women to protect their modesty and save the professors from lecturing to mixed classes. The historian Heinrich von Treitschke, for example, who never permitted women to visit his own Berlin lectures, suggested the creation of "a small medical school for women in some respectable little town."[73] Ludwig Stieda, the professor of anatomy in Königsberg, said he would never teach his subject to coeducational classes but favored separate medical schools for women on the example of the Women's Medical Institute in St. Petersburg.[74] The chancellor of the University of Tübingen recommended parallel courses and institutes within the universities for women studying medicine.[75] A survey of leading German professors in 1897 showed that fourteen out of forty-one with definite opinions on the subject favored the separation of the sexes.[76]

The most compelling responses to suggestions of creating separate schools came from those with actual experience in coeducation. Lydia Rabinowitsch, a native of Russia and former student at Bern and Philadelphia, told the International Women's Congress in 1896 that "to establish special courses for women in Germany, as in Russia or America . . . would [lead] inevitably to universities of the second rank."[77] "All of my colleagues in Germany," wrote Franziska Tiburtius, "agree [that] women doctors do not want separate women's universities." A separately trained woman, she argued, would always be a "second-class physician."[78] Friedrich Erismann, the indefatigable champion of women's study of medicine, cited the many positive reactions of students and professors to coeducation at Swiss universities. This experience, he argued, showed that it was unnecessary and foolish to spend huge sums of money in Germany to build duplicate faculties, clinics, institutes, and laboratories.[79]

In February 1900, the southern state of Baden became the first of the German states to open its universities fully to women. The two universities in Baden, Freiburg and Heidelberg, immediately became the targets of German women seeking full matriculation and degree rights in a university. Four women who had been auditors were immediately enrolled in medicine at Freiburg and another four followed at Heidelberg.[80] Because of the scarcity of gymnasia for women, however, very few could qualify at first for admission. By the summer of 1901, only ten women were matriculated at Freiburg and six at Heidelberg.[81] Gradually, the other German states, pushed by the example of Baden, began to admit women. Bavaria opened its universities to women in 1903, Württemberg in 1904, Saxony in 1906, Hessen and finally Prussia in 1908. In deference to the strong opposition of many professors, the Prussian minister of culture added an important proviso: "Women, with the permission of the minister of culture, can be excluded from individual courses."[82]

The long struggle was over but the guerrilla resistance continued. A number of German professors, especially in Berlin, would not allow women in their classes. Some took all women, some took none, some allowed them in lectures but not in practical instruction. When Abraham Flexner inspected the medical facilities in Berlin, he found a separate dissecting room for women.[83] The medical historian Julius Pagel, who accepted no women in his classes, called their study "one of the perversities of the nineteenth century."[84] Professors Waldeyer and Bergmann announced publicly that they wanted no women in their lectures. An American woman physician in Berlin in 1910 said that even in his public clinics, Bergmann "allowed no female workers or hearers except nurses."[85] In Göttingen, Max Runge wrote: "I am in the position to announce that the director of the Women's Clinic will under *no* circumstances admit women to the obstetrical-gynecological instruction."[86] But the vast majority of professors, whatever their private views, accepted the change quietly and made no effort to treat the women differently. Some, in fact, who had earlier opposed the admission of women to medicine, now commented on their favorable impact on the demeanor of the male students.

## Before the War

With the opening of the great universities of Prussia to women, the number of women training to be physicians rose steadily. Prussian universities enrolled 140 women in medicine in the fall of 1908, 261 two years later, and 416 in the summer of 1914.[87] In all Germany, women's medical enrollment jumped from 312 in 1908 to 1,027 in 1914, or nearly 6 percent of all medical students.[88] As in other countries, medicine was the preferred subject of study of the largest number of women. Because of the lateness of their start, however, few women were actually practicing medicine by 1914. According to the latest figures available before the war, only 138 women were officially counted as practicing physicians.[89]

The first women enrolled in German universities, according to Konrad Jarausch, were quite different from the men who preceded them. As was true in other countries, they tended to be older, less conventionally prepared, more likely to be Jewish, and from more advantaged families than the male students.[90] A considerable number of the aspiring women physicians "had parents or relatives who were both socially prominent and sympathetic to their career aspirations."[91] At least 40 percent of the women students in Germany in 1912, according to a contemporary study, came from academic families. Another study, this time of the women studying medicine in Göttingen in the years 1908–1917, showed 32 percent of them as members of families of higher governmental officials, 26 percent from academic families, and another 26 percent from a merchant background.[92]

The opening of Germany's universities to women brought students from other countries, as had happened in France and Switzerland. The German states, however, were far less open in their welcome to foreign women. Whereas foreign men, including large numbers of Americans and Russians, had been coming to Germany since 1870, the advent of the first foreign women, especially Russians, brought alarm and resistance from the universities. Undoubtedly, the long campaign against the Russian medical women in Zurich in the medical press made the issue a particularly sensitive one. As early as 1899, the students at the University of Halle protested the growing number of foreign women in the medical clinics and demanded that they be excluded. They put out a call to students in other universities to join them in their protest. Although the faculty at Halle disapproved of the students' action, the xenophobia in German universities rose steadily over the next dozen years.[93] Foreign students, both men and women, were made the scapegoats for the general overcrowding in lecture halls and clinics.

Russian nationals and particularly Jews and Poles were made the target of efforts to limit the number of foreigners studying in Germany. "We must keep the male and female Polish students out," wrote Chancellor von Bülow in 1902: "For the Russians, the story is different as long as they do not openly embrace anarchism."[94] At Leipzig, the authorities moved in 1901 to limit the number of Russian women by refusing to accept diplomas from Russian girls' schools for admission. The Prussian ministry of education and the medical faculty at Göttingen took a similar stand.[95] The principal targets of all these actions, write the historians of women's study at Leipzig, were the Jewish women of the Russian empire.[96] As a result, the number of Russian women studying in Germany never reached the levels of Switzerland or France. In 1914, fewer than 150 foreign women were enrolled in medicine in Germany, compared to more than 1,300 foreign men.[97]

The war itself, as in Russia and France, increased the numbers of women studying medicine. The universal need for doctors, along with the declining numbers of men in medical school, encouraged many women to enter the medical profession. By the summer semester of 1918, nearly two thousand German women were studying medicine, or about 10 percent of all medical students.[98] Women physicians served in reserve military hospitals and other war installations. Male medical students with ten semesters of training were drafted as physicians into the military service, but women could be used only as nurses in war areas. A woman who complained about this discrimination was told that to assign a woman as a medical officer would mean giving her officer's rank and "A German man can never be responsible to a woman. That would endanger discipline."[99] Despite their limited role at the front, women doctors earned respect for their work. Former critics now lauded their achievements and self-sacrifice. "For the first time," wrote the gynecologist Fehling of his wartime service, "I used the services of women assistants, and I can offer the best recommendation of their clinical obstetrical activity . . . and their assistance in operations."[100]

For all the resistance and the slowness in opening its universities to women, Germany had made remarkable progress in a short period of time. When the guns sounded in 1914, Germany had passed the United States in the number of women studying medicine, and was second only to Russia in Europe. Switzerland and France, which had for so long been the pioneers in opening their doors to women, had fallen behind. Great Britain, which had taken up the issue of women doctors earlier than most European countries, lagged even further in the rear. On the continent, once women were finally admitted to medical study, and to the strict secondary schools that prepared students for the university, the proportion of women in medicine, even in a nation like Germany that had been adamantly opposed, rose dramatically faster than in Britain or America. It is to the complex developments in the Anglo-American world, including the paradoxical impact of coeducation and the demise of the women's schools, that we turn in the following chapters.

# 6 *The Fight for Coeducation in Britain*

The opening of Germany's universities to women left Great Britain and Russia alone in Europe in their continuing resistance to coeducation in medicine. Switzerland and France, beginning in the 1860s, closely followed by the nations of Scandinavia, the Low Countries, Italy, Spain, and now finally Germany and Austria, had brought women into their universities. In the case of Russia, as we have seen, the women's medical schools would disintegrate in the chaos of World War I and coeducation would become a de facto reality before the Bolshevik seizure of power in 1917.

Across the Atlantic, the United States and Canada, despite the early American lead in opening medicine to women, continued to equivocate on teaching medicine to women in "mixed" classes. "One by one Medical Colleges for men are opening their doors to women as students on an equal footing with men," wrote the editor of the *Woman's Medical Journal* in 1901, but "the experiment is not yet ripe for decisive conclusions." Only the future, concluded the editorial, would determine whether coeducation in medicine would succeed in America.[1] In neighboring Canada, early efforts at coeducation were smashed by faculty and student resistance and separate schools for women were created at Kingston and Toronto in 1883.[2] By the early 1890s, thirteen separate medical colleges for women were being operated in the United States and Canada. When added to the four women's colleges in Great Britain, a total of seventeen medical schools for women only were offering medical instruction in the English-speaking world.

What caused the English-speaking nations, for all their activism in behalf of women, to resist so strongly the teaching of medicine to men and women together in the same classes? Why was even Germany able to achieve full coeducation in medicine before the Anglo-American nations?

Nowhere, certainly, was the doctrine of "separate but equal" education so stoutly defended, often by women themselves, as in the medical worlds of Britain and North America. Separate education was made possible by the relative ease with which private colleges for women as well as men could be chartered by British and American governments compared with continental Europe. Nowhere on the continent could a women's medical college have been created with the legal authority of a London School of Medicine for Women or a Woman's Medical College of Pennsylvania. The women's medical courses in Russia, by contrast, always suffered from their uncertain, extralegal status, which handicapped those who completed them. Furthermore, the pattern of diffused power and responsibility over licensing and practice in Britain made it theoretically possible for a woman doctor to get a license from a qualifying medical body in any part of the kingdom. In the United States, on the other hand, the mere possession of a medical degree (and at times not even that) was all that was necessary to begin the treatment of patients. To become a doctor was simply much easier for a woman in the English-speaking nations than anywhere in Europe.

The continental women made a virtue of necessity. Not being able to create alternative schools, they concentrated their energies on breaking down the barriers to women in the state-run medical schools of their homelands. Once victory was won, it meant inevitably the entrance of women into the same classes as men. It was male educators and physicians, not women, who raised the possibility of women's schools in their last-ditch efforts to thwart the women's movement, and it was women who resisted them. Throughout the continental debate over women doctors, far more attention was paid to academic standards and the fear of creating second-rate physicians than was true in Britain or especially the United States. In the United States, where an uphill battle was still being fought to raise standards in all medical schools, the concern over quality as an argument against separate schools was rarely expressed. "On the European continent," wrote Mary Putnam Jacobi in 1891, "the admission of women to medical schools has depended on the fiat of government bureaus, prepared in this matter to anticipate a popular demand." But in the United States and England, she said, "the movement for such extension of privilege has sprung from the people, it has fought its way,—it has been compelled to root itself in popular sympathy and suffrage."[3]

The strong, early start by American women in a time of universal hostility to female physicians proved eventually a disadvantage to the cause of coeducation. For decades afterward, those seeking to block the entrance of women into the mainstream of medicine were able to point to the women's schools as satisfying the need to provide them opportunities. The schools' very existence enabled critics in America and later in Britain and Canada to reconcile the demands for women's rights of an increasingly democratic age with their personal hostility to teaching and studying in the presence of women. At the same time, they were left free to attack the qualifications of women entering the profession from the large number of weak medical schools that admitted them. "Women were less of a threat in the American medical profession than they were in Europe," writes Martha Hildreth, because of the generally low status of the American profession and the still lower status of women doctors.[4]

What was particularly striking in Britain and America was the considerable number of women who came to prefer the separation of women in medical study. This was especially true of those women who were themselves products of separate medical schools and hospital training. The authors of a study of 430 American women physicians in 1881, for example, after noting that most were graduates of women's schools, concluded that the majority of women students would prefer not to receive all their instruction in mixed classes, "even though this might prove necessary for a first-rate education."[5] Many favored the compromise effected at the University of Michigan, where for eleven years after its medical school was opened to women, professors were paid an extra five hundred dollars per term to teach them in separate classes.[6]

In Canada, a woman who studied briefly in a coeducational school wrote in her diary in 1882 of the torments of study with men: "No one knows or can know what a furnace I am passing through . . . Not because there is anything in the whole range of medicine that should make me blush or feel hurt . . . It is that we are obliged to take it not alone with *gentlemen* but the blackest hearted roughs."[7] Canada soon opted for women's medical schools on the U.S. model. As late as the First World War, a British handbook on "How to Become a

Woman Doctor" advised women that while some students preferred a coeducational medical school, others found "distinct advantages" in a women's school.[8]

But the leaders of the women's medical movement in Britain and North America saw few such advantages. Those women who had experienced coeducation abroad, such as Jex-Blake, Elizabeth Garrett, and Mary Putnam Jacobi, as well as those who had gained entrance to established schools at home, including Elizabeth and Emily Blackwell and Marie Zakrzewska, never wavered in their fight for genuine medical coeducation. The Victorian prudery against mixing men and women in the same medical classes they denounced as largely sham and pretense. For them, separate schools were at best temporary expedients on the way to full assimilation into the medical profession. "Co-education in medicine," wrote Jacobi in 1890, "is essential to the real and permanent success of women in medicine. Isolated groups of women can not maintain the same intellectual standards as are established and maintained by men."[9] In Boston, Zakrzewska continually opposed the creation of a separate school for women, even one allied with Harvard, on the ground "that it would provide the female students with separate and unequal education."[10] In England, Jex-Blake, even after her defeat in Edinburgh, continued to argue strongly for joint education. "Not only in America," she wrote, "has the system of joint education been tried, but at Paris, Zurich, and Bern . . . and friends at each place assure me of the complete success of the experiment, if such it is considered."[11]

The idea of men and women studying and dissecting the human body together in the same lecture halls and at the same tables, however, was particularly sensitive to British and American minds in the high noon of the Victorian era. "In certain subjects," declared Dr. F. W. Campbell of McGill University in 1889, "certain terms have to be employed which certainly could not be used before women without great embarrassment."[12] That they had been used many times in coeducational classes in continental Europe seemed to make no difference. "In Europe," said Mary Putnam Jacobi, "the admission of women . . . has been widely opposed because of disbelief in their intellectual capacity. In America it is less often permitted to doubt—out loud—the intellectual capacity of women. The controversy has therefore shifted to the entirely different ground of decorum."[13] The oft-cited example of coeducation in Swiss and French medical schools, and later those of much of Europe, carried little weight in Anglo-American medical circles. Were not many of the Swiss and French universities' women students, as critics charged, foreigners from different cultures in Eastern Europe and the Russian Empire? Were they not, in comparison with British or American women, insensitive to the requirements of polite society? Only the capitulation of Germany to coeducation caused many to reexamine their position. Germany, after all, was a staunchly conservative, Protestant country, as puritanical in its way as Britain or the United States, and its medical science was the envy of the world.

Even some of women's strongest champions in the United States were skeptical about the wisdom of mixed classes. Both Henry I. Bowditch and James Chadwick of Harvard wanted women to have the chance to study medicine but only in separate classes. "It was his earnest desire," wrote Bowditch's son, "that Harvard University should offer medical instruction to women upon an equal basis with men, but he believed that in many departments separate instruction was desirable."[14] A survey of attitudes among the physicians of Massachusetts in 1878 revealed that of 320 men who favored admitting women to Harvard Medical School, only 127 supported joint classes in all subjects.[15] The *Journal of the American Medical Association*, which had come to accept separate medical schools for women by the 1880s, criticized the University of Colorado for opening its medical school to women. "The co-education of the sexes in medicine," wrote the editor, "has not proved successful elsewhere in this country, and it is doubtful whether it will be possible to maintain it in Colorado without difficulty."[16] Until well into the twentieth century, even in coeducational schools, women were not allowed to attend urology clinics with men.[17]

The women's medical school was therefore the favored institution for training women as physicians in the United States and Canada until almost the end of the century, and even longer in Great Britain. As late as 1894, women's colleges in the United States were still enrolling more than five hundred students of medicine each year.[18] A careful student of women's medical education in Britain estimates that between 80 and 90 percent of all British women qualifying in medicine before 1914 got their principal training in women's schools.[19] Unlike the graduates of America's women schools, however, the British students passed the same examinations for licensure as men and took four or five years to complete their studies.

## The Battle of Edinburgh

In Britain, as in the United States, the separate education of women in medicine came only after excruciating efforts to win admission to the existing schools. As early as 1862, Elizabeth Garrett had been rejected as a student by the University of London and by the Scottish universities. Time and time again, medical faculties in British universities, as in Germany, proved themselves more conservative than colleagues in other fields of university study. When the faculty of London University was confronted with a vote on the admission of women to degree candidacy in 1877, the arts and letters professors voted 80 to 20 in favor of the change and the science faculty concurred 89 to 11, but the medical faculty cast its ballots 21 to 79 against the women.[20]

The struggle to open British universities to women had gone on simultaneously with the harder fight to gain a place for women in medicine. By the late 1860s, a number of girls' schools were preparing students under religious or other private auspices for careers as governesses or teachers. Evening lectures and special classes for women, as in Russia and Germany, were organized in university centers across the nation. The efforts of Emily Davies and others had led to the founding of Girton College for women at Cambridge. A number of the universities, including Cambridge, Durham, and Edinburgh, had opened their local examinations, intended as a measure of secondary-school attainment, to women.[21] But no woman had as yet won the right to matriculate in a British university.

In 1869, Sophia Jex-Blake, who wanted to study medicine, opened a celebrated chapter in British university history at the University of Edinburgh. Her battle to matriculate and graduate in medicine was the most fiercely fought and widely reported event in women's educational history of the nineteenth century. A fiery, determined, and enormously self-confident woman, she rattled the foundations of the conservative educational structure of Great Britain. Those who knew her were agreed on her quick intelligence, inexhaustible energy, and abrasive personality. "Brilliant, hot-tempered and resourceful" was the description of Louisa Martindale, a noted surgeon, who called her "a splendid leader."[22] To Elizabeth Blackwell, she was "a dangerous woman from her power and want of tact," who endangered the movement to create medical opportunities for women.[23] Elizabeth Garrett, somewhat older and more irenic in temperament, found her "overpowering" with "some peculiarities which do not quite harmonize with my own."[24] A later writer would call her "stormy, tumultuous, and unmanageable."[25]

When Jex-Blake left for Edinburgh, she knew that Zurich and Paris had already admitted women and that the American women's schools were open to her. She had spent three years in the United States, where she had worked in Marie Zakrzewska's hospital in Boston, been denied admission to Harvard, and been accepted into the opening class of the Blackwells' medical school in New York. "I don't mean to graduate at any Woman's College—on principle," she had written to her friend Lucy Sewall in Boston.[26] "It seemed to me radically unjust, and most discreditable to Great Britain," she would later write, "that all her daughters who desired a University education should be driven abroad to seek it."[27] Further, she knew that only British licenses or degrees could now be registered under the law. Like Elizabeth Garrett, she had been turned down by the University of London. So, in March 1869, she applied to the University of Edinburgh, which had a reputation for liberalism in matters of education.

Her reception at Edinburgh was at first encouraging. She found support from Sir James Simpson, an old friend and teacher of the Blackwells, and Professor David Masson, who taught rhetoric, as well as from Dean John Balfour of the medical school. Her objective, she told several members of the faculty, was to discover if the school would admit her "given the fact that the precedent had recently been set in Paris and Zurich."[28] She was admitted temporarily by the faculty senate while other bodies in the university considered the matter. Shortly, this action was rescinded by the university court, the highest administrative authority, on the ground of its "not being advisable for the University to make alterations in the interests of one lady." The widespread publicity caused by Jex-Blake's presence in Edinburgh quickly brought four other applicants to the city, including Isabel Thorne and Edith Pechey. Thorne was about to embark for Paris to study medicine when Jex-Blake persuaded her to join the little band of applicants.[29]

A new application by the five women was this time approved by all university authorities with the provision that the women be taught in separate classes. Jex-Blake had already agreed that the women would themselves bear the expense of the extra instruction. "It seemed now," she wrote, "as if smooth water had at length been reached, after seven months of almost incessant struggle."[30] So well did the women students do in their ensuing study that a move was made in the spring of 1870 to abandon the separate classes and spare the women the added expense of their instruction. The women were already paying as much as four times the fees of the male students to some professors. But this effort was narrowly defeated by a group in the faculty led by Thomas Laycock and Robert Christison, who were emerging as the strongest foes of the medical women. Christison's opposition was especially important because he sat on all the governing bodies of the university.

New trouble came with the announcement that Pechey had outscored all of the other first-year students in chemistry. In theory, this entitled her to a Hope Scholarship, which would give her free access to the chemistry laboratory for a period of three months. The professor of chemistry, whose decision it was, yielded to faculty pressure and awarded the prize to a male student on the ground that, having been taught separately, the women were not full members of the class.

Against her own better judgment, Pechey was persuaded by Jex-Blake to appeal the decision. News of the contretemps raised a storm of controversy across England as well as Scotland. Newspapers, journals, and politicians alike joined in the attack on the university and the hapless professor who had made the award (now upheld by the faculty senate). The public attacks on a colleague—in this case, one who had befriended the women—brought dozens of previously indifferent professors into the fray. One friend of the women's cause opined that "their ambition and brilliancy put the cause back fifty years."[31]

Just ahead lay more serious difficulties. In the fall of 1870, the women were to begin their practical work in the Royal Infirmary. The managers of that institution, buffeted by the swirling controversy surrounding the women, were petitioned by the male students to bar their entrance. After weeks of indecision, the managers finally denied them entrance. Emboldened, the men students now determined to keep the women out of the classes in anatomy as well.

Many believed that they were at least tacitly encouraged by professors opposed to female study. On 18 November 1870, they massed before Surgeons' Hall and, after jostling and throwing mud and rotten vegetables at the women, slammed the huge gates of the courtyard in their faces. Inside, according to Jex-Blake, the men were "smoking and passing about bottles of whisky, while they abused us in the foulest possible language."[32] As Isabel Thorne recalled it, "We stood for a few minutes surrounded by the hooting crowd of young men, unable to make our way to the classroom, when a male student rushed from the Hall and opened the gates from the inside."[33] Once in the noisy auditorium, the class was disturbed again by the bleating of a sheep, which had been pushed in through the doors by the protesters. "Let it stay," said the angry professor, "it has more sense than those who sent it here."[34]

The lines were now sharply drawn. Support for the women was dwindling within the university but growing outside. A committee of five hundred citizens was formed to support the women. In a public meeting to elect new managers for the Infirmary, Jex-Blake made a serious error in attacking Professor Christison's assistant as having played a key role in the "Riot" at Surgeons' Hall and in describing the students as only "puppets." "I know," she told several hundred hearers, "that Dr. Christison's class assistant was one of the leading rioters . . . I do not say that Dr. Christison knew of or sanctioned his presence, but I do say that I think he would not have been there, had he thought the doctor would have strongly objected to his presence." Jex-Blake was promptly sued for libel by the assistant. "It took no more than a day or two for the whole country to know," writes Edythe Lutzker, "that her impulsiveness had plunged the little group, and especially Sophia, into a head-on collision with the law."[35] A jury would decide against her but award the complainant only one farthing in damages.

The medical faculty now bent every effort to end the brief experiment in educating women. Without clinical instruction, the women could not graduate. Seven women were now enrolled with no means to complete their education. Although the Infirmary managers were to relent and admit some women in December 1872, the faculty steadfastly refused to grant them a degree. The women, led by Jex-Blake, took the issue to court. When Lord Gifford pronounced in their favor, there was again premature rejoicing among the supporters of women in medicine. But the faculty senate, now unwilling to compromise or admit defeat, appealed the verdict. In June 1873, the Court of Sessions ruled that the decision to admit the women in 1869 had been illegal and that the university had no responsibility to the women. An embittered and exasperated Jex-Blake, reluctant to accept defeat, wrote that "when we came in contact with such unexpected depths of moral grossness and brutality, we had burnt into our minds the strongest possible conviction that . . . women *must,* at any cost, force their way into it, for the sake of their sisters, who might otherwise be left at the mercy of such human brutes as these."[36]

## Why Women Should Not Study with Men

But nearly two decades would pass before another woman would study medicine with men in Great Britain. No British university would consider taking the women of Edinburgh into its student body. Some would finish their degrees at continental universities—Jex-Blake and Edith Pechey at Bern, Agnes McLaren at Montpellier—but future medical women in Britain, as in America earlier, would study medicine only in separate women's schools. It was ironic that Jex-Blake's crusade for coeducation in Edinburgh should end in a movement to found separate schools. All of the other leaders of the women's medical movement in Britain—Elizabeth Blackwell, Elizabeth Garrett, Frances Elizabeth Morgan—blamed Jex-Blake's tactics and fiery temper for the failure at Edinburgh. "Had the same policy of unobtrusively working on, claiming no distinctions, and sedulously and quietly avoiding all occasions of rivalry between the sexes, which led to such marked success at Zurich . . . and in Paris been followed," wrote Morgan in 1884, "the result of the Edinburgh experiment was assured, and years of struggle, heart-burnings, injustice and hope deferred might have been averted."[37]

There was considerable justice in Morgan's charge. The struggle at Edinburgh left a bitter heritage in British medical circles that made further efforts at coeducation nearly impossible. Even when Scotland finally declared for women's higher education in 1889, the medical school at Edinburgh held out against mixed classes until the First World War.[38] Elsewhere in Britain, especially in London, separate medical education for women would remain the rule until well after the war. Abroad, the defeat of medical coeducation in Britain was trumpeted as confirmation of the worst fears of women students in medicine. German writers especially cited the Edinburgh experience to warn their countrymen against repeating the mistake. "With regard to the admission of female students to your University," Wilhelm von Zehender quoted Argyll Robertson of Edinburgh as saying in 1875, "I may be allowed to offer the friendly warning that our experience here is not in favour of their admission."[39]

The dramatic publicity accorded the women's fight in Great Britain gave rise to a new outburst of interest in women's capacity for higher education. At the same time, in the United States, the renewal of the struggle over women at Harvard, and the beginnings of a limited coeducation in medicine at the University of Michigan, forced new attention to women's study there. On both sides of the Atlantic, beginning in the early 1870s, the question of education for women was taken far more seriously than in the preceding decades. In Britain, medical men entered the public debate for the first time. A number of obstetricians and gynecologists warned against the dangers to women's health from excessive study. Particularly effective were the arguments of Henry Maudsley, a professor of medical jurisprudence in London, who borrowed heavily from a Harvard professor, Edward H. Clarke, in attacking the unfitness of women for hard study. The evidence of physiology, claimed both Maudsley and Clarke, pointed to a close connection between physical and mental development. In the case of women, wrote Maudsley, a great deal of energy was diverted in puberty to the organic changes taking place in their bodies. "When Nature spends in one direction," he said, "she must economize in another direction."[40] The strain of intensive study, both warned, was dangerous in a time of great physiological change. "There have been instances," Clarke had written in 1873, of women who had "graduated from school or college excellent scholars, but with undeveloped ovaries. Later they married, and were sterile."[41]

Women, it was now agreed, could perform very well in advanced collegiate work, but only at the expense of normal physical development. Since women needed more rest than men during puberty, especially during menstruation, they needed a different, less strenuous, kind of education. "The regimen of a college arranged for boys, if imposed on girls," wrote Clarke, would foster a whole host of debilitating diseases.[42] If women were to be educated at all, according to many medical men in Britain and America, it should be only in separate schools arranged according to their needs. The strenuous mental and physical demands of medical study and practice should particularly be avoided if a woman expected to marry and lead a normal life. "I confess that I have been surprised in America," wrote Jex-Blake after a trip to the United States, "to find how much study young women do seem to accomplish without material injury."[43]

The import of the Maudsley-Clarke arguments for separate education was clear. Women's schools, if properly arranged, were far better for women than coeducational schools. Even if taught separately, however, women must think long and clearly about the effects of intensive study on their lives. The offensive against coeducation, especially in medicine, when added to the defeat at Edinburgh, made new efforts to open medical schools to women discouraging at best. Women themselves accepted much of the biological determinism of the separatist champions. It fitted well with the older argument for women doctors as particularly suited to treat women patients.[44] At Ann Arbor, where women were taught in separate classes in the "coeducational" medical school, Clarke's book was eagerly read by women as well as men. In addition, "the president and the faculty read it, and shook their heads doubtfully about the 'experiment in coeducation.'"[45] At the University of Maryland, a professor charged that "too much brain-work and too little body-work" had produced "a host of sickly girls who swarm in every class of society." Dozens of women's diseases, "mostly of uterine complexion," were spawned in the recitation room. "To redeem woman from the bondage of her education and restore her to wifehood and motherhood," he concluded, "these must be the great missions of the physician."[46]

## A Women's School in London

In Britain, the ranks of medical educators and practitioners closed against any further attempts at coeducation. Public opinion, which had been outraged by the treatment of the women at Edinburgh, cooled toward the idea of common classes. Many influential Londoners who had supported the cause of Jex-Blake and her little band now joined in the effort to create a women's medical school in the city. The women who became students at the new school, writes Elizabeth Fee, "were treated as a special and peculiar group, and were inundated with anxious advice. They were cautioned not to indulge in extreme views but to preserve their womanly virtues, to submit voluntarily to strict discipline, to join literary and athletic clubs, to eat enough, [and] to avoid anxiety."[47]

Jex-Blake was again the leading spirit in the London venture. This time, however, she was forced to play a less public role as more influential and better-connected women, such as Elizabeth Garrett and Elizabeth Blackwell, were drawn into the enterprise. Both of the older women had reservations about launching a separate school. Graduates of such a school, Garrett warned, "would at once be marked as a special class of practitioners, subordinate and inferior to the ordinary doctor." Better that women should go to Paris, she wrote in a letter to the *Times,* where they could get a first-rate education comparable to any man's. Jex-Blake responded angrily, "protesting as strongly as lies in my power against this idea of sending abroad every Englishwoman who wishes to study medicine."[48] Blackwell likewise was reluctant to join with Jex-Blake—"this belligerent woman"—but did agree to join the organizing council. "I now seem compelled to step in," she wrote, "for my experience and judgment can supply the control [that is needed]."[49]

It was Jex-Blake, however, whose drive and determination made the school a reality. Her "impetuosity," according to a later historian, "was largely responsible for the swiftness with which an idea was made a fact."[50] Money was raised, a house was rented, and a faculty was found to teach the courses. Critical help came from Dr. David Anstie, who had told Jex-Blake in December 1873, that "your best course would be to take some premises in London and build a thoroughly good school, fit for first-class teaching . . . I believe if that were done, you would get the teachers."[51] Once the school was launched, Anstie counseled, one or another of the nineteen official examining boards in the kingdom would admit its students to candidacy. Encouragement came, too, from such notable medical and scientific figures as Burdon Sanderson, Hughlings Jackson, and Thomas Huxley, all of whom agreed to serve on the provisional council of the school.

When Anstie died suddenly, just before the opening of the school —Jex-Blake called his death "a terrible calamity"—the anatomist

A. T. Norton was persuaded to become the first dean.[52] Fourteen students, twelve of them from Edinburgh, made up the first class as the school opened quietly on 12 October 1874. In the course of the year, nine more students enrolled. Since the income from student fees fell short of expenses, a fund-raising campaign was begun in London and Edinburgh.[53]

More serious were the lack of clinical instruction and the uncertain future of the school's graduates. No London hospital would open its doors to women students, and without acceptance by one of Britain's examining bodies no graduate could gain official recognition as a practitioner. For several years, beginning in 1872, Parliament had alternately raised and lowered the hopes of women that a legal remedy was at hand. Finally, in 1876, a bill was approved "enabling" but not requiring examination boards to admit women to candidacy. Not until the liberal Irish College of Physicians and the Queen's University of Ireland agreed to admit women to examinations and diplomas later in the year was a way opened to grant women an official license to practice. This, said Jex-Blake, was "the turning point of the whole struggle." The final hurdle was passed in 1877 when the Royal Free Hospital agreed to admit women medical students to its wards. A few months later, the University of London voted, over the opposition of its medical faculty, to open all its degrees to women.[54]

The school grew very slowly in its first years of existence. Only six new students entered in 1875, two in 1876, and nine in 1877. The requirements for admission kept many away: a knowledge of botany, chemistry, history, English, modern geography, Latin, arithmetic and algebra, the first two books of Euclid, and a modern foreign language.[55] In 1883, Elizabeth Garrett Anderson replaced Norton as dean. Jex-Blake had protested the appointment, believing that it was Garrett Anderson who had prevented her from playing a larger role at the school. Three years later, Jex-Blake started her own women's medical school in Edinburgh, widening the breach with her London comrades.[56] The London school became increasingly interested during the 1880s in training women for medical missionary work.[57] By 1890, it enrolled more than a hundred women, and its former students accounted for over 90 percent of all the women listed in the British Medical Register. Yet some women continued to take their medical degrees abroad, for reasons of prestige and lesser cost, after preparing themselves in London. At least 32 of the 106 women registered in 1890 held degrees from Paris, Bern, Zurich, or Brussels. Most of the women physicians serving on the Board of Governors of the school had in fact taken degrees in foreign universities.[58]

A woman surgeon who studied at the school in the 1890s recalled that "the amenities were not great." The dissecting room, she remembered, was divided by a curtain; on one side were held the anatomy lectures, on the other, the " 'subjects' we were to dissect after the first three weeks of lectures." Other facilities were equally makeshift. Lectures in physiology were held in "a very chilly room" built in the garden, while the chemistry laboratory "was a poor one." But she praised the teachers, who, by this time, included a number of women.[59]

## New Openings for Women

The range of opportunities for British women to study medicine widened in the thirty years before the First World War. Although the London School continued to lead in the enrollment of women, new women's schools were opened in Edinburgh, Dublin, and Glasgow, and a number of the established universities began to drop their bans on female study. The women's school in Edinburgh, called "excessively reliant" on Sophia Jex-Blake by one historian, lasted only twelve years after its founding in 1886. Her single-minded approach to educational problems alienated many in the Scottish capital, as it had in London. A rival women's school, which survived until World War I, was launched in opposition. The most successful of the women's schools outside London was that in Glasgow. Here, in 1890, a school of medicine for women was opened at Queen Margaret College, soon to be a part of the University of Glasgow. The founding of the medical school came just a year after Parliament had opened all of the Scottish universities to women, which meant that Queen Margaret deliberately chose to follow a segregated pattern of education. Many of its students, reports the historian of its medical school, "were subsequently to regret this decision." Arguments about mixed instruction in medical subjects continued to plague the school until long after all other teaching had become coeducational. When the first medical classes were offered at Queen Margaret under university auspices in 1892, fifty women took their places. The number rose gradually to 109 students on the eve of World War I.[60]

One interesting aspect of the Glasgow school was its appeal to women from somewhat less affluent families. Almost all of the early students who accompanied Jex-Blake to Edinburgh or enrolled at the London School of Medicine for Women had of necessity come from comfortable families of the middle and upper classes. At Glasgow, by contrast, a significant number of the women studying were the daughters of skilled workers, shopkeepers, and small farmers, although the large majority came from professional and commercial families as in London. The somewhat wider appeal of the Glasgow school has been attributed to the lower costs of Scottish medical education and the special tuition grants made available by Andrew Carnegie after 1901.[61]

The opening of the Scottish universities to women was an important extension of opportunities for British women in medicine. It was a victory for women's groups in Scotland, who, together with liberal-minded professors, had long campaigned for the reform. The Act of 1889 was followed by three years of preparation before women were actually admitted in 1892.[62] The medical schools at St. Andrews and Aberdeen opted immediately for mixed classes, while Glasgow, as we have seen, and Edinburgh, remembering the great battles fought a decade before, chose to teach women in separate courses. As in Prussia, the new law exempted those professors still opposed to coeducation from teaching women in their classes.[63] At first, few women seized the new opportunities to study medicine. A single woman joined 268 other medical students at Aberdeen in 1895; two years later, another lone woman began her solitary way through medical school before committing suicide soon after graduation.[64] At St. Andrews, a new school of medicine, opened in 1898, attracted only six women to its first class.[65] Even where medical schools were opened to women, however, dissecting rooms remained largely segregated.[66]

In the ancient school of Edinburgh, according to a modern historian, "the backlash from the stormy years of the Jex-Blake period discriminated most against the medical women students."[67] Women were allowed to graduate from the university in medicine but were forced to take instruction at one of the two women's schools still operating in the city. The Royal Infirmary, which had remained closed to women until 1892, now gave them instruction in separate wards from men.[68] Fewer than ten women studied medicine at the

university in the years before 1900.[69] When Abraham Flexner visited
the city in 1912, he found the instruction and facilities for women
notably weaker than elsewhere in Scotland. "It must be admitted,"
he wrote, "that the Edinburgh authorities appear to no slight extent
to be governed in their position by hostility to co-education in medicine."[70] It was not until 1916 that women in Edinburgh were taught
in the same classrooms and facilities with men.[71]

Meanwhile, outside London, a number of the civic or "red brick"
universities had also begun to add women to their classes. As in
some of the Scottish universities, the women who went to the recently founded universities in Birmingham, Bristol, Durham, Leeds,
Liverpool, and Manchester came in larger numbers from the lower-
middle and working classes of England. Coeducation quickly became
the rule in most of the classes, and little of the controversy surrounding women in medical school was heard in these cities.[72] The changing mood toward medical education in these provincial cities was
evident in the ease with which a motion was defeated at Owens
College in Manchester in 1899 to send women "to other available
institutions." By a vote of twenty-one to two, the Senate agreed with
Principal Adolphus Ward that the whole purpose of the college was
to allow students to "obtain [education] at home without expensive
resort to distant seats of learning."[73] Of course, medicine played a
distinctly smaller role and its teachers were far less influential in
these schools than in those of London or the older universities.

In the years before the First World War, the opposition to medical
coeducation gradually eased. The success of common classes in Scotland and in the civic universities made the question less controversial
than in the early days at Edinburgh. The war itself gave a strong
push to the efforts to end segregation in medical teaching. But even
in 1914, after a half-century of hard struggle, the most prestigious
schools of Britain at Oxford and Cambridge were closed to them.
Nor had any of the twelve medical schools of London, with the
exception of the school for women, moved to allow women into
their ranks. "Women entered medical education," writes Mary Ann
Elston, "under a limited mandate which shaped their training, their
access to professional institutions and their career opportunities."[74]
The schools that were open to women, furthermore, educated far
fewer physicians than did those of France, Germany, Switzerland,
Russia, or the United States. As the war began, fewer than five

hundred women were enrolled in medicine throughout Britain.[75] Those who graduated encountered the same obstacles to getting an internship or a hospital appointment as women in the United States and Canada.[76] By and large, the cause of coeducation in medical training in 1914 was considerably less advanced in Britain than in any other major country.

# 7 *America: Triumph and Paradox*

The same ambiguity about women's special traits and fitness for medicine that was so influential in Great Britain lay deep in American and Canadian attitudes toward the woman doctor. On the one hand, the women's medical movement in North America insisted on broadened and equal opportunities for medical study; on the other, it acknowledged that women were different from men and that special arrangements for their study might be necessary. "Feminism rarely led them to challenge accepted Victorian definitions of femininity," writes Regina Morantz-Sanchez of women physicians in the United States; "they infrequently opposed the concept of separate sexual spheres, arguing instead that women had a role in medicine by virtue of their special qualities of nurturance, which would both compensate for and be complementary to the role and achievements of men." The argument for a special place in medicine for women was readily translated into a justification of special schools for women. Separate schools, in turn, suffered from their isolation from the mainstream of medicine. The resulting stigma of inferiority, says Morantz-Sanchez, "was internalized if not perpetuated by women doctors themselves."[1]

## Coeducation and Separatism

Both coeducation and separate schools for women were more widespread in the United States than in either Britain or Canada. European critics often saw coeducation itself, especially in the primary and secondary schools, as largely an American phenomenon. "The two features of American education . . . which strike an Englishman as characteristic," wrote Jex-Blake in 1867, "are the union of all classes in the same schools, and of both sexes in the same colleges."[2] By 1900, all but 2 percent of American public schools were coeducational, and a growing majority of colleges and universities were admitting women. "The American people," said Nicholas Murray Butler of Columbia University in 1902, "have settled the matter."[3] Yet at the same time a considerable number of separate colleges, including those in medicine, were being created for women, especially in the eastern states. By 1910, three out of five colleges and universities in the United States were coeducational, while 15 percent of them were open to women only.[4]

In Canada, women's education was growing more slowly than in the United States. Canadian women were more strongly influenced by the British example than by events south of the border. The women's movement in Canada, Käthe Schirmacher observed, was less vigorous than that in either England or the United States. As late as 1912, she wrote, "the study and practice of medicine [in Canada] is made very difficult for women."[5] Canadian women began coming south to American women's schools as early as 1867, when Emily Stowe graduated from the homeopathic New York Medical College and Hospital for Women. Eight years later, Jennie Trout finished her studies at the Woman's Medical College of Pennsylvania. On their return to Canada, both women faced a "chill reception" from Canadian authorities and the medical profession.[6]

The years after 1870 were, in general, a time of slow and uncertain growth in the medical education of women in North America. Much of the earlier opposition to female doctors had abated in the United States, but coeducation, especially at first, made only slow and halting advances. Some women found their way into public clinics and hospitals for training but more were still dependent for clinical instruction on women's hospitals and dispensaries. Teaching in the women's colleges was gradually improving, and some women were now numbered among their faculties, but change was gradual and resistance to women in positions of authority stubborn. "Comparisons are often made between the opportunities offered to medical women now, and 25 years ago," Marie Zakrzewska told her interns and staff in 1883, "but there is still very little opportunity for women to learn *from women.*"[7]

Prior to 1880, thirteen regular schools of medicine were open to women in the United States. Of these, the schools in Philadelphia, New York, and Chicago were for women only. A number of the western state universities, particularly those in Iowa and Michigan, were now allowing women to enter their medical classes, but the numbers were usually small and the programs often weak. The small medical school of the State University of Iowa, for example, was coeducational from its very first session in 1870, when it admitted eight women. In the first twenty years of its existence, only forty women were graduated in medicine.[8] Of all the state universities, Michigan was the best known, the largest, and the most respected. Its decision in 1870 to admit women was hailed as the beginning of real coeducation in medical training in the United States.

For twelve years, the regents of the University of Michigan had wrestled with the issue of coeducation. A survey they had made of other colleges and universities had brought an avalanche of negative counsel. President James Walker of Harvard, for example, told them that "there is an immense preponderance of enlightened public opinion against this experiment." From Yale, President Theodore Woolsey wrote that he was "averse to mingling the sexes in any place of education above the school for the elements." Even the president of coeducational Antioch College, Horace Mann, warned that while "the advantages of a joint education are very great[,] the dangers of it are *terrible.*" The state's press joined in the growing controversy. Coeducation, said the Detroit *Free Press,* "would tend to unwoman the woman and unman the man." Public pressure for allowing women into the university continued to grow, however. In 1867, the state legislature, more liberal and cost-conscious than the university, declared for a policy of coeducation at Ann Arbor. But even after the regents made their final decision in 1870 the medical faculty stubbornly resisted. They petitioned the regents for an exception to the coeducational policy in the case of medicine. The matters discussed in their classes, they wrote, were far too delicate for women to hear in the presence of men. If they must teach women, they asserted in a last-ditch defense, it should be in separate classes and for extra remuneration. The regents yielded on both points. Only George Willard, who had championed the women's cause, voted against the arrangement, arguing that "women could properly be admitted to most medical lectures in common with male students."[9]

Michigan thus became the first prominent university outside Europe to accept women on a continuing basis in medicine. Of the thirty-three women who came to Ann Arbor in the fall of 1870, eighteen enrolled in medicine. A number of them came from distant states to take advantage of the new chance to study medicine. From New York, for example, came Amanda Sanford, a graduate of the Woman's College of Pennsylvania, who would receive the university's first degree in medicine. When word of Michigan's action reached the staff of the New England Hospital in Boston, Eliza Mosher recalled, five women in the laboratory abandoned "their seemly demeanor . . . joined hands and danced about the laboratory table." Mosher would later become the first dean of women at the University of Michigan.[10]

Enrollments in medicine at Michigan grew steadily. By the end of the decade, forty-three women were studying in the medical school and twenty-six had graduated.[11] President James Angell, who took office as coeducation began, defended what he continued to call the "experiment" to colleagues across the country. In an indirect reply to the defender of separate schools, Edward Clarke, Angell wrote in 1879 that after nine years of experience with coeducation, "the solicitude concerning the health of the women has not proved well-founded. On the contrary, I am convinced that a young woman, coming here in fair health, . . . is quite as likely to be in good health at the time of her graduation as she would have been if she remained at home."[12]

In a surprisingly short time, the Ann Arbor school became the premier institution for educating women in medicine in the United States. By 1881, more than 20 percent of the entering medical students were women. In that year, the faculty finally asked to end the separation of the sexes that had caused them to repeat every lecture and demonstration for the benefit of the women. The Regents agreed to allow each professor to make the decision for his own class. "In some cases," according to one account, "the walls originally segregating the sexes diminished into curtains behind which the women could hear the lectures without being seen by the men." Other classes, notably anatomy, continued to be taught separately. Still others were demarcated by a red line on the floor of the classroom, which separated the women's places from those of the men. At least some lectures were segregated in this fashion until the end of the century.[13]

The school in Ann Arbor was responsible for the graduation of nearly a hundred women doctors by 1900.[14] In the meantime, after 1880, fourteen more of the regular medical colleges throughout the country had moved to admit women. Citing the example of Michigan, an encouraged Marie Zakrzewska wrote that "I think it impossible to work for the elevation of the standard of [women's] medical education in any other way than by having the leading women of each state keep in view as their final aim the opening on the basis of coeducation of the best medical colleges."[15]

## Coeducation Slowly Advances

But the education of women in mixed classes proceeded very slowly. In 1870, the women in Ann Arbor and Iowa City were almost alone among American and Canadian women in studying medicine in a university medical school. Women's schools and sectarian colleges, as they had since 1850, continued to account for the large majority of all women graduates throughout the 1870s and 1880s. By 1890, when Scotland was opening all its universities to women, American women's schools still enrolled two-thirds of all the women studying medicine in the United States. Only 257 women of perhaps a thousand enrolled in all types of medical schools in the United States were studying in a coeducational regular college.[16] In Cleveland alone, schools of homeopathy were responsible for 80 percent of all the medical degrees earned by women to 1914.[17]

The battle for coeducation in medicine was fought in dozens of states and scores of medical colleges in the last three decades of the nineteenth century. Even in the irregular schools, women were sometimes barred by faculties opposed to mixed classes. The Eclectic Medical College of Pennsylvania, for example, which operated from 1850 to 1880, listed no woman among its matriculated students.[18] The Penn Medical College, on the other hand, established separate sessions for women, arguing that coeducation had been tried "and proved unsatisfactory to both teacher and pupil."[19] A homeopathic school in Cincinnati, the Pulte Medical College, debated the issue strenuously for seven years before cautiously deciding for coeducation. In reaching its decision, the faculty sought the advice of colleagues in other colleges of homeopathy. By the time of their survey in 1878, the homeopathic institutions in Boston, Cleveland, Iowa City, Ann Arbor, and two schools in Chicago were all admitting women. The dean of Boston University's school reported that he was "entirely in favor of mixed classes"; a colleague in Cleveland said that the presence of women was a "restraint on rudeness, boorishness and vulgarity"; while a faculty member of the homeopathic school in Iowa City admitted that "it is rather embarrassing to treat on delicate subjects before a mixed class."[20] Later, a homeopathic college in Baltimore would welcome women into its first class in 1891.[21]

At Harvard, a new effort to bring women into the medical school was narrowly beaten back by its opponents. "For vehemence and personal animosity almost resulting in disaster," wrote an early historian of Harvard Medical School, "no recent controversy equals that . . . over the admission of women" to the school.[22] At one point, the whole faculty was at the point of resigning en masse. It began with a letter from Marian Hovey in 1878, offering the Medical School $10,000 "if its advantages can be offered to women on equal terms with men." A joint committee of overseers and medical school faculty members under the chairmanship of Alexander Agassiz recommended that a trial be made. The committee rejected, however, the evidence of coeducational experience in Europe and America as "inconclusive." In Europe, read the report, "the social conditions are so far different from those in America that the experience of the former does not apply to the latter."[23] In a private letter to Mary Putnam Jacobi, Agassiz referred to the frictions with male students "which have closed Edinburgh Med. School for women and which have made so much trouble in Zurich." On the European practice of teaching the most delicate subjects in mixed classes, he told her: "It may be that hereafter we may come to accept such an association as most natural, but with our present ideas, no matter how good a spirit may be brought to such mixed classes, the objections natural to most people still persist as they are inherent in the thing itself."[24] The committee nevertheless favored a trial, with separate classes in most subjects. "It looks as if Harvard would really admit women," wrote Francis Minot of the medical school, following release of the committee's report.[25]

But the medical faculty, by a vote of thirteen to five, promptly disavowed the report. The reason given was the extensive changes then under way in the school, which made "the experiment in admitting female students" inexpedient. In the face of the opposition of the faculty, the "generous proposal" of Marian Hovey was declined. Opposition to admitting women, said Agassiz in 1879, was now stronger than six months before.[26] A medical journal opined that "Harvard has had a narrow escape."[27] Two years later, a committee of women led by Marie Zakrzewska offered Harvard $50,000 to allow women into its medical school. Again, the medical faculty protested, by an even larger vote, that "female medical education cannot be undertaken in the Medical School without a serious risk of detriment to the interests of the medical education now given to men."[28]

Elsewhere, women were here and there admitted to regular medical classes in a number of the western states in the 1870s and 1880s. In 1876, the first woman physician graduated from the University of California. During the next decade, Cooper Medical College and the University of Southern California were also educating women in medicine.[29] One California school, presumably the University of California, excluded women students from its surgical and venereal wards, according to a contemporary letter, "not by law but by public sentiment." A number of the professors, the letter continued, "are much opposed to the women studying with the other students and will try to have the privilege withdrawn on the ground of morality."[30] East of the Rockies, the University of Colorado began a policy of coeducation when it opened its medical school in 1883.[31] Other western and midwestern states were also enrolling a small number of medical women in their public universities by the middle of the 1880s.

In Canada, change came even more slowly. A decision at Queen's University in Kingston to take a few women in 1879 as an experiment brought three women into a special course in medicine the following year. After one year of special lectures, the women were allowed to join the men's classes in October 1881. They were given a separate dissecting room, however, and "for awkward lectures, like obstetrics and medical jurisprudence, they sat in a little room adjacent to the general classroom so that any embarrassed blushes would go unnoticed by the young men." The professor of physiology, however, turned his classroom into a continuing attack on the presence of the women. Male students were given "every opportunity to be lewd and rude and crude." When the women walked out after one particularly offensive outburst, the men responded with an ultimatum: either the women must be expelled, or all the male students would move en masse to Trinity Medical School in Toronto. In a one-sided compromise, the women were allowed to finish their studies but no more women would be allowed into the college.[32] Thus ended the first try at medical coeducation in Canada.

The failure of coeducation at Queen's led to the creation in 1883 of two women's medical schools in Kingston and Toronto. At Kingston, Jennie Trout, who had graduated from the Woman's Medical School of Pennsylvania, played a key role in organizing a women's school in loose affiliation with Queen's University. "The College is as much as possible a WOMAN'S COLLEGE," read an early catalogue, "and a student coming here can, from the moment she enters the city, have the advice and interest of ladies."[33] In its ten years of existence, the Women's Medical College graduated thirty-four physicians.[34] More ambitious was the Toronto enterprise, where Emily Stowe, whose daughter had suffered acute embarrassment as the only woman allowed to study medicine in another short-lived experiment, won a good deal of support from the male establishment. Within six years, the Woman's Medical College of Toronto was enrolling thirty-five students in its four-year curriculum.[35] At the time of its merger with the medical school of the University of Toronto in 1906, 112 women had received their M.D. degrees from the college.[36] This represented more than half of all the medical degrees awarded to women in Canada to that time.

The continuing resistance to coeducation in Canada and the United States and the grudging admission of only a few women to American public universities made the women's medical college the principal resource for most women. Even after Michigan and other state schools had begun to enroll women, new women's schools continued to appear to meet the growing need. Between 1870 and 1890, no fewer than twelve new women's medical schools were founded in the United States and Canada. They were located in Chicago, New York, Baltimore, St. Louis (2), Atlanta, Cincinnati (2), Kansas City (2), and the two in Canada.[37] In addition, the older women's schools in Philadelphia and New York continued to offer instruction. Some of the newer schools were short-lived, such as the homeopathic school in St. Louis; others later merged, as was the case with the two schools in Cincinnati; and still others, like the Woman's Medical College of Chicago, became part of coeducational universities. By 1899, only eight of the women's schools survived.

Almost all of those that survived were now regular schools. After the demise of the homeopathic school in St. Louis in 1884, only the New York Medical College and Hospital for Women, founded in 1863, remained of the earlier irregular colleges for women. This homeopathic school would be responsible for graduating 382 women physicians in the years before 1914.[38] The remaining regular schools were of varying size and strength. The Woman's Medical College of St. Louis, for example, was founded in 1891 and enrolled about thirty students each year until its demise in 1896.[39] In Kansas City, a women's school that opened in 1895 boasted a faculty drawn largely from the University of Kansas School of Medicine but enrolled few students.[40] Cincinnati, according to a local physician, somewhat exaggeratedly, had "at least three women's colleges" in 1893, "and it is not easy to ascertain facts regarding them."[41] One of the Cincinnati schools was the subject of a letter to Mary Putnam Jacobi, describing it as "one of the unpardonable sins against a confiding public."[42] Another was run by the Presbyterian Hospital in Cincinnati, which by 1894 enrolled thirty-five students and had graduated fifteen women physicians.[43] This school merged with the Woman's Medical College of Cincinnati the following year, and the successor college graduated fifty-eight more women before it closed its doors in 1903.[44]

By far the weakest of the women's schools, at least as seen through its announcements, was the Woman's Medical College of Atlanta, Georgia. To be admitted to the college, officials announced in 1889, an applicant need be only "of good moral character, have fair education, and be not less than 18 years old." A year later, eighteen students were taking classes in the school and seven were scheduled to graduate. The course of study was five months, including a Christmas recess. As to dissecting, "the faculty would gladly dispense with this branch, which is a 'bugbear' to every lady student, but conscientious teaching will not permit."[45]

The strongest of the schools for women were those founded earlier in Philadelphia, New York, Chicago, and Baltimore. The Woman's

Medical College of Pennsylvania, in particular, had become the leader among them because of its early start, capable leadership, and staunch local support. Of all the schools, it attracted students from the largest number of states and foreign countries. Alumnae files show registrations from twenty foreign countries and nearly every state. From Canada alone came thirty-three women, beginning with Emiline Wolverton in 1852; twenty-four came from India; seventeen from Russia; and fourteen from England. The ubiquitous Russians included Adelaide Lukanina, who came from Zurich in 1875, and a number of Jewish women barred from expanding opportunities at home.[46] Files of the college also contain a letter from an English-woman who had been with Jex-Blake at Edinburgh, and who had then studied in Paris and worked in India, before applying at age fifty-six to enter the Philadelphia school.[47] Forty-five of the graduates of the college were serving as medical missionaries by 1907.[48] The college was notable, too, for the number of southern women who came north to study medicine in a women's school. A partial list includes the names of eighteen women from eight southern states.[49]

The women's schools in New York, Chicago, and Baltimore were also popular among women interested in medicine. All of them, as was true of Philadelphia, listed a number of women on their faculties, some of them with experience in laboratory research and foreign study. At the New York school, for example, Anna Williams, a student of the late 1880s, left an account in her unpublished autobiography of learning chemistry from a French woman named Chevalier, of being initiated into bacteriology by the Zurich-trained Anna Kuhnow, and of her dissecting experience in "the horribly fascinating study of Anatomy." She described Mary Putnam Jacobi as a "short, energetic-looking" woman who "made many of the students feel uncomfortable by her clever manner of showing how much we needed to learn."[50] Farther west, Mary Thompson was able to recruit a strong faculty for her Chicago school that included such well-known women as Eliza Root, Marie Mergler, and Bertha Van Hoosen. All of them had had some experience abroad. Thompson herself built a reputation as the best woman surgeon and teacher of surgery in the Middle West.[51] Meanwhile, in Baltimore, the Woman's Medical College, begun in 1882, benefited from the attention of a number of the famous professors at the new Johns Hopkins University School of Medicine, as well as from support from the local profession. Among its teaching faculty in 1898 were five women, one of them, Claribel Cone, a full professor of pathology.[52]

Student life in the women's colleges was rigorous and controlled, though less strict than the closely supervised lives of medical women in Russia or Britain. The women in Philadelphia heard formal lectures every day of the week, including Saturdays, and twice a week took a long ride on a horse-drawn streetcar to the clinics of the Blockley or Pennsylvania hospitals. They lived together in boarding houses near the college, where their lives were notably freer than those of their sisters in London or Leningrad. The course of study by 1881 was graded by subject and lasted three years for those who had not completed an apprenticeship with a practicing physician. The women still wore long skirts, flowing blouses, hats, and gloves to their classes.[53]

Most of the graduates of the women's schools went on to practice their profession. A survey in 1881 of American women physicians, most of them products of women's schools, revealed that 390 of 430 women responding were in active practice. Well over half had been active for more than five years. The average age of the women when starting to practice was thirty-one and a half years. More than 90 percent said that menstruation had never interfered with their work. In fifteen states, they had become members of state or county medical societies. Only sixty-five of the women had married since graduation—a lower percentage than in either Britain or Russia—but some had been already married when beginning medical school.[54]

A more detailed survey of twenty women graduating from the Woman's Medical College of Pennsylvania in 1879 showed similar results. The average age of the graduates was thirty (three were over forty); eleven of them were married (three to physicians); six had been teachers before entering medical school; and only two had been to college. Especially interesting in this survey was the considerably larger number of women than in Europe who came from less affluent families. Four of the twenty had fathers who were farmers, and seven came from families where the father was an artisan or a tradesman.[55] Yet the surveys also revealed, as Virginia Drachman has demonstrated, how segregated the lives of women physicians in America continued to be. "Women doctors," she writes, "were still studying in women's medical schools, training in women's hospitals, caring almost exclusively for female patients, and tending not to join professional medical societies."[56]

Black women, most of them from middle-class families, were occasionally found in the women's schools after the Civil War. The first black woman to graduate from a medical school, Rebecca Lee, had earned her medical degree from the New England Female Medical College in Boston even before the war ended. The women's schools in Philadelphia and New York then graduated the second and third black women physicians in 1867 and 1870.[57] By 1900, according to a list compiled by Bettina Aptheker, sixty-one black women had completed their studies in medicine in the United States, forty-four of them at Howard University and Meharry Medical College, both coeducational schools, and eleven at women's colleges, nine of them at the Woman's Medical College of Pennsylvania.[58] Most of these early black women physicians came from families who, "perhaps to protect them from menial labor or domestic servitude, encouraged their daughters to educate themselves." Educated black women of the nineteenth century had even fewer job options than white women, but medicine, along with teaching and nursing, lay open to the talented and ambitious.[59] As late as 1920, however, only sixty-five black women were actually practicing medicine, or fewer than one percent of the women in the profession.[60]

From the founding of the first women's school in Philadelphia in 1850 to the outbreak of war in Europe in 1914, more than twenty-nine hundred women graduated from the five principal U.S. women's medical colleges, including the homeopathic school in New York (Table 6). Another four or five hundred, it can be estimated, won their degrees in the short-lived women's schools in other cities. Until well into the twentieth century, they were responsible for the majority of women graduates in active medical practice in the United States and Canada.

## The Demise of the Women's Schools

Not until 1894 did coeducation finally overtake separation in American medical education. A year after the opening of the much-heralded medical school at the Johns Hopkins University to both men and women in 1893, 878 women were studying medicine in classes shared with men, while 541 were enrolled in schools for women only. Attendance at women's schools then fell sharply for the rest of the decade and reached 183 by 1904. More and more of

*Table 6.*   Graduates of principal women's medical colleges, 1850–1915

| School | Number of graduates | Period covered |
|---|---|---|
| Woman's Medical College of Pennsylvania | 1,420 | 1850–1914 |
| Woman's Medical College of Chicago | 575 | 1870–1902 |
| Women's Medical College of the New York Infirmary | 422 | 1868–1899 |
| New York Medical College and Hospital for Women | 382 | 1863–1914 |
| Woman's Medical College of Baltimore | 120 | 1882–1910 |

*Sources:* "Deceased Alumnae," *Register of the Alumnae Association of the Woman's Medical College of Pennsylvania, 1850–1970,* pp. 109–127; Anon., "Woman's Hospital Medical College, Woman's Medical College of Chicago," MS, Northwestern University Woman's Medical College Records, Archives and Special Collections, MS-112, p. 3; Woman's Medical College of the New York Infirmary, *Final Report,* pp. 25–33; printed list of graduates of New York Medical College and Hospital for Women, source unknown, Archives and Special Collections; Abraham, *Extinct Medical Schools of Baltimore,* pp. 119–125.

the previously segregated men's schools dropped their bars against women. Where only thirty-five medical schools, fewer than half of them nonsectarian, were open to women in 1890, ninety-six schools were coeducational a decade and a half later.[61] By that time, only three women's schools remained in operation (those in Philadelphia and Baltimore, and the homeopathic college in New York), and the number of schools closed to women had dropped to sixty.[62]

What had happened? For one thing, the training of physicians had undergone a dramatic change since 1870. Pressures were intense to extend the period of study, screen applicants more carefully, equip laboratories, and add new subjects to the curriculum. Medical teaching in the United States and Canada was becoming increasingly individualized, time-consuming, laboratory-oriented, and enormously expensive. State after state began to raise requirements for the licensing of physicians. The organized profession itself began to work more effectively to raise standards in medical education. More and more, it made little sense to try to operate a school of medicine outside the confines of a sheltering university. Those medical colleges that were sustained largely by student fees, a group that included all of the women's schools, found themselves in a constant struggle to maintain reasonable standards and still remain open. One by one, the women's colleges, like dozens of other independent and weakly financed schools, began to close their doors.

Other factors contributed to the demise of the women's medical schools. The steady growth of coeducation itself, especially in the public universities, made it increasingly difficult for the private colleges to maintain their barriers against women. By the 1890s, furthermore, more than five thousand women were engaged in medical practice in the United States, and many had been admitted to state and county medical societies. Their growing presence and influence in the profession could no longer be ignored. Each step toward the assimilation of women into the mainstream of medicine made weaker the defense of educational separatism. Enlightened doctors were aware, too, of the world trend toward coeducation in medicine. Only Russia and Germany, both widely viewed by Americans as reactionary and autocratic, still held out in Europe against attempts to bring women into universities, and there were signs that Germany was beginning to crack.

The capitulation of a great private university, Johns Hopkins, to medical coeducation was a symbolic event of the greatest importance. No university had enjoyed such favorable public attention for its efforts to open a premier institution for medical training in America. Its early professors, hired long before the start of medical instruction, were known widely across the country. Its standards, laboratories, and well-endowed hospital were something new in the American experience. When, therefore, the trustees, acutely aware of the staggering costs of the venture, accepted the gift of $500,000 from a group of women on condition that women be admitted, their action was hailed as the dawn of a new era. "The fiat has gone forth [from] Baltimore," wrote Mary Putnam Jacobi, that "it is not immodest for women to study anatomy and physiology together with men."[63] The aging Emily Blackwell, uncertain about the future of her own school in New York, said: "When a college of the standing of Johns Hopkins received women on equal terms, we felt that a great step in advance had been taken."[64]

It was at first argued by the women's committee soliciting funds for the school that the opening of Johns Hopkins would not "take

the place of the medical schools for women" but instead "will afford
to women in America those opportunities for advanced medical
training which they are at present compelled to seek in the great
foreign schools of Vienna, Paris, and Switzerland."[65] But it soon
became clear that the much-publicized action of the Baltimore school
would have far-reaching effects across the country and in Canada.
"Since the Johns Hopkins has set the pace," Sarah Hackett Stevenson
told an international gathering of women in 1893, "the least that
the inferior universities and schools can do is to follow after as fast
as possible." On the basis of economy and justice alone, she said,
"co-education is desirable."[66] For all of the reasons given, dozens of
medical colleges began to broaden their entering classes to include
women, while the women's schools felt the pressure of the unac-
customed competition.

By 1900, opportunities for coeducational study were opening
everywhere. Cornell University followed the example of Johns Hopkins in accepting women in medicine in 1899. The medical schools
in upstate New York in Buffalo and Syracuse were already open to
women. Three of Boston's four medical schools were now accepting
women. Farther west, a half-dozen medical colleges in Chicago were
competing for female as well as male students. In St. Louis, the Barnes
Medical College opened to women in 1900. Colorado and California
each had three medical schools serving women by 1900. In Oregon,
Michigan, and Kansas, women in the state universities accounted
for more than 20 percent of all medical students. The Omaha Medical
College in Nebraska was graduating a small number of women each
year by 1900. In Kentucky, a homeopathic and a black medical
school allowed women to enter. In Canada, as we have seen, the
University of Toronto began accepting women in its regular medical
classes in 1906. Other Canadian medical schools had opened to
women earlier. Of the older, established private schools in Canada
and the United States, only McGill, Pennsylvania, Yale, and Columbia remained closed to women until the First World War, and Harvard until 1945.[67]

The abrupt shift to coeducation, together with the new standards
and the enormous cost of medical teaching, caused most of the wom-
en's schools to shut their doors. The schools in Atlanta, St. Louis,
Kansas City, Cincinnati, and Toronto were all gone by 1903. Of the
four strongest of the regular schools, only the women's college in

Philadelphia survived to 1914. The school founded by the Blackwells in New York was the first of the well-known colleges to go. In 1899, as Cornell declared its willingness to admit women, Emily Blackwell and her trustees faced the inevitable and ended the school's thirty-one-year career. "The friends who established, and have supported, the Infirmary and its College," Blackwell told the last graduating class, "have always regarded co-education as the final stage in the medical education of women." Now, she said, "medical education may hereafter be obtained by women in New York in the same classes, under the same faculty, with the same clinical opportunities, as men."[68]

The next women's college to fail was in Chicago. The school founded by Mary Thompson had reached a peak of enrollment in the early 1890s, registering 152 students, when it affiliated with Northwestern University. Northwestern had committed itself to continue the women's school as a separate entity. Faculty members believed that access to Northwestern's "extensive physiological and pathological laboratories" would help greatly in keeping the school's standards high. Soon, however, enrollment at the Chicago school began to plummet, reaching a low of nine entering students in 1899.[69] By this time, six other medical schools in Chicago were admitting women and the competition was intense. The budget deficit at the women's school reached $10,000 dollars in 1900, and Northwestern began considering its options. "Unless satisfactory arrangements [can] be made with the present faculty of the Woman's Medical School," read a report from a special university committee, "this School [shall] be permanently closed."[70] Two years later, the school was abruptly terminated with no provision made for its students. Bertha Van Hoosen, who had just begun teaching gynecology at the school, read the news in the local newspaper. "As in an earthquake," she wrote, "the earth had opened and the Northwestern University Woman's Medical School had disappeared."[71] In an ironic twist, Northwestern proceeded to bar women from its male medical school until 1926.

By 1910, only the schools in Baltimore and Philadelphia, as well as the homeopathic college in New York, remained of the dozen women's schools of twenty years before. In that year, Abraham Flexner gave relatively high marks to all of the women's schools in his famous report for the Carnegie Foundation for the Advancement of

Teaching. The New York Medical College and Hospital for Women was described as having laboratories that were "attractive and well kept," while its equipment was "simple, but recent." The Baltimore school, he reported, had "small laboratories" that were "scrupulously well kept," but the clinical facilities for students were "quite insufficient." In Philadelphia, the Woman's Medical College of Pennsylvania had "intelligently equipped and conscientiously used" laboratories. He paid the college an unusual compliment by calling attention to the "striking evidence of a genuine effort to do the best possible with limited resources." Yet none of the schools, he argued, "can be sufficiently strengthened without an enormous outlay."[72]

The schools in Baltimore and Philadelphia were already in deep trouble when Flexner arrived. Within a month of his visit, the dean of the Baltimore school was writing to his counterpart in Philadelphia that "we are considering closing our college" and asking whether the Woman's Medical College of Pennsylvania could take the remaining twelve students.[73] At the final commencement, President Guy L. Hunner explained that inadequate funding, too few students, and the inability to meet the new requirements of the American Medical Association were responsible for the closing.[74]

Meanwhile, in Philadelphia, Dean Clara Marshall faced the worst crisis in the school's threescore years. Enrollment had dropped 25 percent since 1900 and was still falling. The disappearance of the other women's colleges caused many to question whether the school was still needed. Efforts were made, without success, to find an affiliation with another medical school. Flexner himself was approached to seek his help in getting foundation support, but he was adamant in his opposition to the separate medical education of women.[75]

To make matters worse, the college was threatened in 1913 with loss of its "A" rating by the American Medical Association. The secretary of the Association's Council on Medical Education, N. P. Colwell, wrote Dean Marshall that the needs of the college were "quite serious" and remedial action was required. Among other complaints, Colwell listed the "bare legal minimum requirement" for admission, the small number of "expert, full-time, salaried professors," the shortage of clinical material and equipment, and the lack of any real medical research.[76] Another inspection the same year added to the list of concerns. "It seems a pity," the report concluded, "that finances should not be forthcoming to insure the continuance of at least one good medical school which is strictly for women students."[77] Still the school "limped along," in Regina Morantz-Sanchez's phrase, bolstered by the conviction that coeducation had not solved all women's problems and helped by the intransigence of Philadelphia's other medical schools to admitting women.[78] This school alone would survive the turbulent era and remain a women's college for another sixty years. The homeopathic college in New York, on the other hand, expired in 1918.

## Success and Disappointment

The swing toward coeducation convinced most women that the battle for acceptance in medicine was nearly won. More than 80 percent of all women studying medicine in the United States and Canada were in coeducational schools by 1910. Access to schools of the highest quality, in the opinion of Sarah Hackett Stevenson, "has forever established the status of training of the woman doctor in the United States."[79] Separatism as a strategy for women's advancement was clearly on the wane. The end of the women's schools, in the opinion of Mary Putnam Jacobi, meant an end to the low standards and mediocrity that had marked instruction at most of the women's colleges.[80] The changes wrought in women's position in medicine seemed decisive and final. The Russian Lydia Rabinowitsch, who had taught at the Woman's Medical College of Pennsylvania and was now working with Robert Koch in Berlin, told a women's group in 1897 that the women doctors of America could serve as models for their European sisters. "It is really an enviable life," she said, "that many of our American sisters lead."[81]

But the road ahead was strewn with obstacles. The sectarian and women's schools—tolerated but never accepted by the now triumphant regular profession—formed an uncertain heritage on which to build for the future. Some of the most prestigious American and Canadian schools and hospitals, moreover, continued to bar women; a few still relegated them to separate classes. Some schools that had opened to women, such as Georgetown and George Washington universities, ended the experiment in coeducation in the 1890s.[82] Across the country, as Lynn Gordon has demonstrated, educators

were having second thoughts about coeducation and looking for
ways to channel women into domestic and nonscientific studies.[83]
At the University of Iowa, women's medical enrollment declined in
both the homeopathic and the regular medical schools.[84] Hospital
appointments as interns or residents, because of the continuing
doubts about women and the freedom of private institutions to dis-
criminate, were always far more difficult for women to attain than
for men. Many of the most desirable of the emerging specialties—
often controlled by private boards—became nearly exclusively male
in the years ahead. More important, the rapidly rising standards for
admission to medical school, the increasing costs of medical education, and the simultaneous shrinking of the number of places in
the fewer medical schools made a career in medicine more rather
than less difficult in the early twentieth century.

Enrollment of women in medical schools in the United States
dropped precipitously from 1,280 in 1902 to 526 in 1913. At Michigan, the proportion of women in the medical school fell from a peak
of nearly 20 percent to only 5 percent in 1910.[85] The Kansas Medical
College, whose student body was 31 percent female in 1893, had
only 4 percent women among its students in 1907.[86] More often
than men, women lacked the opportunity for a thorough premedical
education and generous family support. Only two hundred of America's women doctors at the end of the century, according to the
educational historian Thomas Woody, had had college training.[87]
The strictures of N. P. Colwell against the low admissions standards
at the women's college in Philadelphia were indicative of a widespread problem. Further, new occupations were opening to women
by the early twentieth century that required less educational preparation and shorter periods of training than medicine.

The ironic result of the social and scientific changes that had rocked
medical education in North America was a diminution of women's
role in it. Across the Atlantic, by contrast, no corresponding decrease
in the number of places in the government-run medical schools or
sudden raising of premedical requirements or tuition costs to the
student affected the women of Europe. On the contrary, once women
were finally admitted by law to medical study—as had happened in
most of Europe—and to the strict secondary schools that prepared
students for the university, the proportion of women, as we have
seen, rose dramatically faster than in the United States or Canada.

The decimation of a generation of young men in war undoubtedly added to the educational advantages of European women. Only in Great Britain did the rate of change lag in the prewar period.

The structural looseness of the American profession, which had permitted weakly supported women's as well as men's medical colleges to flourish under private control, enabled private interests to continue to exert enormous influence even into the twentieth century. In Europe, especially on the continent, the far greater involvement of government ensured that women in medicine, once the political struggle was won, would approach equality of treatment and participation. Students of women's medical education in the United States have stressed the attitudinal obstacles to women's full participation in medicine—and they were undeniably strong—but have not sufficiently noticed the equal or stronger attitudinal resistance to women's study in Europe. The frequently cited writings of E. H. Clarke, for example, which undoubtedly had an enduring effect on American thinking, pale before the stony resistance and rigid denigration of women's capacities in the work of Robert Christison, Theodor Bischoff, and P. J. Möbius. It was the laissez-faire structure of American medicine, so long the despair of reformers and the subject of ridicule by Europeans, that made change so difficult and its effects so uneven.

Even the much-vaunted numbers of women practicing medicine in the United States before 1914 need to be reexamined. "A large number of the women recorded in the census tables," observed Mary Putnam Jacobi in 1891, "will not be found among the graduates of any suitable colleges, or on the registered lists of regular physicians."[88] Jex-Blake, when she surveyed American women physicians in 1886, reported that only 470 women were known to have taken a regular medical degree.[89] The French scholar Caroline Schultze, attempting to compare American with European graduates, published a figure of 1,925 graduate women physicians in the United States in her 1889 study. Of these, according to her breakdown, 580 were regular graduates, 139 homeopaths, 460 "specialists in obstetrics" (midwives?), and the rest divided among other "specialists."[90] In 1900, the alumnae of the Woman's Medical College of Pennsylvania were asked to determine the number of women physicians practicing in the states where they lived. In the twenty-four states, including all of the larger states, for which a report was made, somewhat more than 1,800 women were counted.[91] A reasonable estimate of graduate women physicians, both regular and irregular, in 1900, when the census recorded 7,399 women doctors, would be somewhere between 3,000 and 3,500.[92] Such a figure belies the oft-cited reports of a huge number of trained women around 1900 and begins to bear some resemblance to the data on women medical graduates in Europe. It also makes less dramatic the decline in women's medical enrollment after that time.

In America as in Britain, the outbreak of war in 1914 marked a new acceptance of women doctors in a time of national need. Hundreds of women served in medical units in the armies of Great Britain, Canada, and the United States. Fifty-five women were employed as contract surgeons in the United States Army alone.[93] For many medical women, as Ellen More writes, the war "represented an opportunity for professional assimilation."[94] Graduates of the Woman's Medical College in Philadelphia in 1915, according to a reporter, "expressed a wish today to go to Europe and serve as doctors on the battlefield."[95] The shortage of interns and residents opened new places to women in hospitals. The first women residents were admitted to several hospitals in Philadelphia in 1915, and the Massachusetts General Hospital appointed its first woman intern at the end of the war.[96]

In Britain, the devastating effect of the war on medical schools caused three of the London schools, at least temporarily, to open their clinics to women.[97] The number of women studying medicine rose dramatically. "Any effort which aims at the training of medical women," the London School of Medicine for Women announced, "has thus become of increased importance to the nation."[98] By 1918, twenty medical schools in Great Britain and Ireland were accepting women students, and the enrollment of women had surpassed that of the United States for the first time.[99] "It was in these years," declared Christine Murrell, "that the public for the first time became accustomed to the woman doctor, and ceased to regard her as a freak."[100]

The long years of striving seemed nearly over. To medical women of the early twentieth century, the changes in their lifetimes had brought them within reach of a cherished goal: to study and practice medicine on terms of full equality with men. In looking back, Mary

Putnam Jacobi reminded them of the painful costs of the struggle they had waged:[101]

> It [the struggle] has been fought, and modestly, in the teeth of the most painful invective that can ever be addressed to women,—that of immodesty. Girls have been hissed and stampeded out of hospital wards and amphitheaters where the suffering patient was a woman, and properly claiming the presence of members of her own sex; or where, still more inconsistently, non-medical female nurses were tolerated and welcomed. Women students have been cheated of their time and money, by those paid to instruct them; they have been led into fields of promise, to find only a vanishing mirage. At what sacrifices have they struggled to obtain the elusive prize! They have starved on half rations, shivered in cold rooms, or been poisoned in badly ventilated ones; they have borne a triple load of ignorance, poverty, and ill health; when they were not permitted to walk, they have crept,—where they could not take, they have begged; they have gleaned like Ruth among the harvesters for the scantiest crumbs of knowledge, and been thankful. To work their way through the prescribed term of studies, they have resorted to innumerable devices,—taught school, edited newspapers, nursed sick people, given massage, worked till they could scrape a few dollars together, expended that in study,—then stepped aside for a while to earn more. After graduating, the struggle has continued,—but here the resource of taking lodgers has often tided over the difficult time.
>
> These homely struggles,—the necessity in the absence of State aid, of constantly developing popular support and sympathy for the maintenance of the colleges and hospitals, has given a solidity, a vitality to the movement, which has gone far toward compensating its quaint inadequacies and inconsistencies.

# Epilogue: Since 1914

The long journey to acceptance for medical study had taken women by 1914 almost literally to the ends of the earth. Beginning with Elizabeth Blackwell, women from all parts of the world had repeatedly been forced to leave home, family, occasionally children, and often country to find a place in a school of medicine. Blackwell herself had left her home in Cincinnati to study with sympathetic tutors in North Carolina and Philadelphia, then journeyed to the country medical school in Geneva, New York, and finally left America for the great hospitals of Paris and London. The young Englishwoman Sophia Jex-Blake had spent three years of her life in the United States gaining hospital experience not available at home before undertaking her great crusade in Edinburgh and then finishing her studies in Switzerland. From distant Kazan, eight hundred miles east of Moscow, the revolutionary Vera Figner had traveled across her homeland, then through Eastern and Central Europe, to reach the medical oasis of Zurich. Her countrywoman Adelaide Lukanina spent two months crossing Europe and the Atlantic Ocean in 1875 in order to study at the Woman's Medical College of Pennsylvania. The redoubtable Franziska Tiburtius left her island home in the Baltic Sea to travel south across her German homeland to find a haven in Switzerland. From the Indian port of Calcutta, the youthful Ananhaibai Joshee, who had less than four years to live, set out on 7 April 1883 to sail halfway around the earth to become the first of a number of Indian women to enroll in the Woman's Medical College of Pennsylvania.

The picture that emerges across the intervening years of these determined women is of hundreds, at times thousands, of women in unceasing motion, their lives marked by struggle, suffering, and disappointment, and constantly engaged in a conflict with social expectations and established custom.

Nor had the battle been fully won even in 1914. The Great War that burst upon Europe did bring unprecedented opportunities and a smashing of barriers to medical study in nearly every country. The women physicians of Britain, Russia, and Germany, in particular, reached new levels of acceptance in the terrible devastation of war. At the staid University of Marburg, German women made up 30 percent of all medical students by 1917; in the British medical school in Manchester, the number of women students shot up 400 percent between 1914 and 1918; and in revolutionary Russia, the women's medical courses at Leningrad were abruptly thrown open to a flood of 1,426 new students, men as well as women, in 1918.[1] By war's end, more than ten thousand women were studying medicine in these three countries alone. The ill wind of war, said the editor of the *Medical Woman's Journal,* "brought much good to medical women in that it opened so many schools to women students and so many hospitals to women internes."[2] The demographic catastrophe of war had affected a whole generation of European men and made easier the subsequent broadening of economic opportunity for thousands of women.

Inevitably, as the guns were stilled, the reaction came. Men of the warring nations were given a sympathetic reception as they returned from military service to medical school or training hospital. Competing women were accused of "taking the places" of the returning veterans. Women at Aberdeen were blamed for lowering the quality of university degrees during the men's absence in wartime.[3] The chairman of London Hospital's board, Lord Knutsford, declared in 1922 that his hospital, now that the crisis had passed, would take no more women students. "It has been found," he said, "that the difficulties in the way of providing an adequate medical education at a mixed school are insurmountable."[4] The University of London had already moved to limit the number of women admitted to medical study.[5] In Germany, likewise, a strong reaction was felt against the huge growth in female medical study during the war. "Women doctors," according to one account, "became at once second-class physicians as soon as the question came up of the distribution of

scarce study places, assistant positions, and state insurance patients."[6] The proportion of women in German medical schools
dropped 17 percent between 1923 and 1928.[7]

In the United States, a similar reaction, though weaker, set in.
Since the period of American engagement in the war was brief and
the casualties far fewer, the effects on medical education and the
supply of physicians were less drastic. Nevertheless, the demand for
additional doctors for the military and the effect of male enlistments
on the medical schools were real. A dozen medical colleges, including
some of the nation's most prestigious, brought women into their
medical classes for the first time during the war. Even Harvard flirted
briefly in 1917 with the idea of accepting women to replace the men
lost to military service. The number of women studying medicine in
the United States, which had been declining, leaped from a low of
592 in 1915 to 818 in 1920.[8] Once the war was over, however, the
pressures for change diminished and some began to regret the actions
taken in wartime. At the University of Pennsylvania, for example,
which had only recently begun to admit women, the senior medical
class voted in 1920 to oppose continuing the practice, saying that it
"disadvantages every student."[9] By this time, women were caught
up in the national conservative reaction to the changes of wartime
and the Progressive Era.

Only in the Soviet Union did access to medical training for women
improve immediately in the postwar years. Women had taken an
important part in the war and the revolution, and in the struggle
against Bolshevism's enemies after 1918. "The image of the revolutionary woman as the tough-willed equal of men," writes Richard
Stites, "deepened in the crucible of this bloody war."[10] The medical
schools, as we have seen, had been thrown open to all comers in
1918. Women flocked in growing numbers into the crowded classrooms. In the new social structure built by the Soviets, women were
given by law an equal educational status with men. The woman
doctor was glamorized by state propagandists as vital to the public
health of the nation. Within a short time, women became a majority
in Soviet medical schools; they reached the 70 percent level by 1934.
At the same time, the prestige of the healing professions dropped
in comparison with the technical and entrepreneurial occupations,
which were now more highly valued in a rapidly industrializing
society.[11]

   In the rest of Europe, the proportion of women in medicine, following the setbacks of the postwar era, began to climb once more
in the late 1920s and 1930s. By 1929, the number of German and
Austrian women in medical school had regained the levels of 1920.
French women learning medicine passed the three thousand mark
by the same year.[12] Other nations, including Spain, Switzerland,
Belgium, and Greece, showed substantial increases in the enrollment
of women in their medical schools.[13]

   In Great Britain, however, old doubts about coeducation continued
to plague women in the immediate postwar years. Although Oxford
University conferred its first medical degree upon a woman in 1922,
the situation in London, where most practitioners were trained, remained threatening to women's interests. One by one, the schools
and hospitals that had admitted women in wartime closed their doors
to them in the 1920s. By the end of the decade, only the London
School of Medicine for Women and the University College Hospital,
which admitted only twelve women each year, were teaching
women students in London. "The main reason for the exclusion of
the women students," explained the British correspondent of the
*Journal of the American Medical Association*, "was the objection of men
students to coeducation."[14]

   A report to the senate of the University of London in 1929 stated
that "with few exceptions, the authorities of the medical schools
appear to be convinced that men, if they have a choice, prefer to go
to schools that do not admit women." The committee nevertheless
declared that it "is unable to see any valid argument against the
provision of coeducation in medicine," but stopped short of urging
the complete opening of London's schools. Instead, the committee
recommended irenically that there should be three types of clinical
education in the city: schools for women (that is, the London School
of Medicine for Women), mixed schools, and schools for men only.
The senate gave its approval to the report and "resolved to invite
those schools not at present admitting women to consider the possibility of admitting a quota." Not until 1948, however, was the
invitation fully accepted and single-sex medical education in London
ended.

   The role of powerful private interests in thwarting medical coeducation in London was matched in many of the private schools and
hospitals of America in the 1920s and 1930s. So long as the force

of law was limited in its application to private discrimination, the
degree of societal acceptance of women in medicine would not approach that of continental Europe. Since the 1860s, governments in
Switzerland and France had given women the legal right to study
medicine in all their medical schools; much of continental Europe
had followed by 1914; and now the Bolshevist state had decreed the
equality of women in all its schools and universities. Even those
states, such as Germany, where private hostility to women doctors
remained high, now easily surpassed the United States in the proportion of women in medical schools and hospitals. Although Europe
and America shared similar gender conventions about women's role
in medicine, it was the relationship of medical education to the state
that proved to be the most significant factor in determining women's
success. When state control held private prejudices in check, women
benefited; when institutions and licensing were more privatized,
women often lost out in a complex but discernible way.

In America, in any case, the continuing resistance of a number of
elitist schools to admitting women, along with the restrictive policies
followed by many private hospitals and associations, limited the
victory that medical women had won over discrimination and separatism. The fight to enter medical school and then get an internship
in Europe, as we have seen, was long and bitter, but, once won, it
was over. American women had to fight a thousand different battles
on a variety of terrains to win the same advantages as a single political
victory in Paris or Berlin. As late as 1934, 28 percent of American
medical schools, despite eighty years of agitation, had not yet graduated a single woman physician.[15] Only 99 of 696 hospitals offering
approved internships, furthermore, had thrown open their compe-
titions to women applicants.[16] Women's hospitals still accounted for
a significant number of the women being given clinical training.
"What would the women students of the past eighty years have
done," asked Kate Hurd-Mead in 1933, "without such segregated
hospitals in which to study?"[17]

The policies of hundreds of private boards, hospitals, and training
institutions in the United States and Canada reinforced the continuing prejudice against women doctors in the years between the wars.
Why were so few women entering medicine? "The reason," said
Bertha Van Hoosen in 1930, "is the same as our pioneer great-
grandmothers had to face"—the medical schools and hospitals "sim-

ply don't want them."[18] The weakening of the women's movement in the 1920s, furthermore, left no powerful voice, private or public, to counter the remaining restrictions on women's right to prepare for and practice medicine.

Other reasons can be found, of course, for the decline of women's participation in medicine during these years. Some scholars have pointed to the undeniable changes in women's lives in the United States and Canada, especially the attraction of other professions and occupations, and the shift in gender relations toward a marital model of woman-as-mate.[19] Others have stressed the continuing discrimination and hostility of individual educators, counselors, and physicians against women physicians as limiting factors.[20] Still others, claiming that there was no outright discrimination against women in medical schools, have insisted that the reasons for the American decline must lie in the women themselves.[21] What such explanations overlook, however, is that these same changes in gender relations, opening of new occupations to women, and continuing personal prejudice against women doctors were also found in Europe, where the proportion of women in medicine rose during the interwar years.

More significant in explaining the failure of the medical women's movement in America, following its period of greatest triumphs, was almost certainly the prolix and private character of much of the medical, hospital, and licensing structure that served the American profession. Left to themselves, unchecked by government or powerful political forces, private interests were able to perpetuate in ways both open and subtle an all-pervasive, nagging perception of women's unsuitability for medical practice. When challenged, they cited the availability of other places for women, especially in public institutions, or the high cost of reconverting hospital facilities for women residents. Medical schools justified their limited number of women students by pointing to the example of other schools, and the generally low level of women applicants. "I am a bit skeptical as to the real value" of encouraging women to apply, wrote Dean William Pepper of the University of Pennsylvania to Hans Zinsser of the Harvard Medical School in 1926; "my present feeling would be that we might admit each year to our First Year Class which numbers 110 some three or four women." This opinion, wrote Pepper, "is for your information and it is not for publication."[22] Many women of the period came themselves to believe, as had their predecessors half a century before, that only the truly dedicated and exceptional woman should or could compete for the increasingly scarce positions in medical school or hospital. Women, it was widely affirmed, were too apt to "drop out" of their studies, to marry, to become pregnant, or otherwise to waste the scarce training resources of an increasingly scientific profession.

For some women the earlier years of easy access to study, numerous women's schools, and more relaxed standards seemed in retrospect like a golden age. Some blamed the loss of the women's schools for the sharp decline of the number of women preparing to become doctors. Others called for a new commitment to the remaining separate women's institutions. But the schools and hospitals for women had been themselves a badge of separation and hence inferiority from the first. To be sure, some of them, as scholars have since argued, were for a period as strong as most of the men's schools and hospitals in their preparation of physicians. But after 1900 only those institutions could survive that were prepared for the spectacular increases in the costs necessary to meet the rapidly changing standards of state licensing boards and the profession itself. Efforts to combine the new scientific and professional orientation of medicine with the older gender separation of the nineteenth century were doomed to failure. "The attempted amalgamation of modern, scientific professionalization and Victorian social feminism," writes Ellen More, "was untenable."[23]

By the 1930s, in any case, the American failure was increasingly clear. The proportion of women in medical school scarcely rose above 5 percent throughout the decade. Meanwhile, in Europe, the numbers of women studying medicine had risen sharply in many countries. In Germany, for example, women accounted for one-fifth of all medical enrollment in 1932–33. More than six thousand German women were preparing to be doctors, or more than six times the number in the United States.[24] Even in Britain, the proportion of women completing medical school and listed on the Medical Register by the middle of the 1930s was double that of their American counterparts. In the 1930s and 1940s, according to one study, women doctors in Great Britain increased in number by 237 percent.[25]

The Great Depression and the Second World War brought renewed upheaval to all social groups in industrial society, including women doctors. In many countries, there was a marked hostility to women's competing for jobs with men in the years of economic chaos. In Germany, the Nazi regime quickly dissolved the existing women's organizations and moved to limit women's access to the universities and the professions. The proportion of women in the German universities dropped from 16 percent in 1931 to 11 percent in 1938.[26] In the first year of National Socialism alone, the number of women entering medical school fell from 1,118 to 871.[27] Alice Hamilton, after a visit to Germany, wrote in 1934: "German women had a long and hard fight but they had won a fair measure of equality . . . Now all seems to be lost and suddenly they are set back, perhaps as much as a hundred years."[28]

Hitler's war, however, like the war a quarter-century before, stimulated a huge new demand for doctors in Germany and all the belligerent states. The mobilization of civilian populations on an unprecedented scale across Europe brought thousands of women into professional and technical careers for the first time. Hundreds of thousands of casualties in all the major countries created a sharp demand for physicians and health personnel. By the end of the war, a quarter or more of all the medical students in France, Germany, and Britain were women, while the proportion of women among those studying medicine in the Soviet Union had reached 80 percent. In the United States, less severely affected by the war, the medical enrollment of women increased more slowly, reaching the level of 8 percent in 1945.[29] Several of the remaining private medical schools closed to women in the United States and Canada finally opened their entering classes to women. Citing the "spirit of the time" and recognizing "the wonderful work women are now doing in Europe," the Hahnemann Medical College of Philadelphia admitted women in 1941 for the first time in its ninety-three-year history.[30] Four years later, as the American war effort depleted the medical school of men, the Board of Overseers at Harvard approved a recommendation to admit women.[31] Hospitals, too, began accepting women as interns and residents in ever larger numbers. "Hospitals are hanging out the welcome signs to women physicians these days," said the *New York Times* in 1942; "fledgling women doctors, once excluded . . . are now being snapped up as fast as the ink dries on their diplomas."[32]

The patterns of women's medical education set before 1914 were still clearly visible in the post–World War II world. After 1945 Russia, followed by Poland and at some distance by Germany and France, continued to offer women of the major nations the fullest opportunities to become physicians. In the 1960s about 75 percent of Russian physicians (as opposed to specialists) were women, while in Poland women accounted for 45 percent of the country's graduating doctors, followed by Germany at 30 percent, France and Holland at 20 percent, Italy at 19 percent, Sweden at 17 percent, and Switzerland at 14 percent.[33] Great Britain, in many ways, had made the greatest progress since 1914. Not only were the London medical schools finally opened to women after the war, but the University Grants Committee, supported by postwar governments, began to put pressure on universities to admit more women to their medical schools. By 1966, 25 percent of Great Britain's medical graduates were women.[34]

In the rest of Europe, two of the nations of Eastern Europe that had sent large numbers of their women westward to learn medicine before the First World War, Bulgaria and Yugoslavia, now had medical schools made up of 30 percent women students. Beyond Europe, a number of the nations of Asia, notably the Philippines, Indonesia, Thailand, India, and Korea, were enrolling 20 percent or more women in their colleges of medicine.[35]

Only the United States seemed stalled amid this worldwide change. Here the trend toward fewer women in medicine, first observed before 1914, continued with small fluctuations in the years after 1945. The numbers of women in medical school, which had grown during World War II, fell to a postwar low of 1,463 in 1953. During the 1950s and 1960s women accounted for 5 to 8 percent of medical students and did not reach 9 percent until 1969–70. "Only South Vietnam, Madagascar, and Spain," lamented one analyst in 1971, "have proportionately fewer women in medicine."[36]

Not until the 1970s—more than a century after Mary Putnam and Susan Dimock had won their degrees in Paris and Zurich—did American women begin to gain a place in their own schools and hospitals that rivaled that of Europe. The renaissance in women's medical study owed much to the new women's movement of the late 1960s and its willingness to use powerful legal and political measures, as well as to the simultaneous opening of thousands of new places in America's expanding medical schools and hospitals. A class action suit brought in 1970 by the Women's Equity Action League against every medical school in the nation was instrumental in promoting change. The full force of government was finally brought to bear in scores of affirmative action and antidiscrimination cases across the country. The heavy dependence of medical schools and hospitals on government support made them more vulnerable than ever before. In a single year, the medical schools of Boston doubled their enrollment of women students.[37] National enrollment of women climbed steeply through the 1970s and 1980s. By 1990, women accounted for 36 percent of all medical school enrollment in the United States, and the proportion was still climbing. The number of places won by women interns and residents likewise doubled and then tripled in a short period. In Canada, the medical enrollment of women rose even more swiftly, reaching 44 percent in 1990.[38]

A similar rapid growth took place in Britain and the other nations of Europe. By the end of the 1980s, nearly half of those entering medical school in Britain, once the laggard among European nations, were female.[39] In France, writers were describing the changes in that country by 1989 as the "feminization" of the health professions.[40] Germany by the early 1990s was graduating more than two women doctors for every three male graduates.[41] Similar changes, less dramatic, were reported in other European states and in other parts of the world.

The new women doctors, as described by surveys in several countries in the 1980s, were more likely than men to see their profession as a humane vocation, to be less interested in its pecuniary rewards, and to concentrate in such specialties as internal medicine, pediatrics, and general practice. More than their predecessors, the women physicians at the end of the twentieth century were apt to marry, to remain in active practice, and to carry on their work in a hospital-based clinic.[42] More significantly, perhaps, the old prejudices against women in medicine had begun to fade as their numbers approached near equality with men in a growing number of medical schools.

Although critics continued to worry that new misfortunes might befall the medical women's movement, as they had so often in the past, the mood of the early 1990s was clearly optimistic that the battles of the past would not have to be refought. The changes wrought in medical institutions and public perceptions, after a century and a half of daunting struggle, seemed this time to be final and lasting.

# Notes

*Prologue: 1871*

1. The principal source of information about Mary Putnam's studies in Paris is her published letters in Ruth Putnam, ed., *Life and Letters of Mary Putnam Jacobi* (New York: G. P. Putnam's Sons, 1925). The quotation from the letter to her mother is on page 169. See, too, Rhoda Truax, *The Doctors Jacobi* (Boston: Little, Brown, 1952). The record of her formal admission to medical study in Paris is a letter from the vice-rector to the dean of medicine, 4 June 1868, in her student dossier in the Archives Nationales, Paris.
2. Reprinted in Putnam, *Life and Letters*, pp. 290–291.
3. Faculté de Médecine de Paris, Relevé des Inscriptions, Mlle. Putnam, Mary, Mary Putnam dossier, Archives Nationales.
4. Haryett Fontanges, *Les femmes docteurs en médecine des tous les pays*, 3rd ed. (Paris: Alliance Coopérative du Livre, 1901), pp. 36–37.
5. This account is based on Victor Böhmert, *Das Studieren der Frauen mit besonderer Rücksicht auf das Studium der Medicin* (Leipzig: Otto Wigand, 1872), p. 4, and Hanny Rohner, *Die ersten 30 Jahre des medizinischen Frauenstudiums an der Universität Zürich, 1867–1897* (Zurich: Juris Druck & Verlag, 1972), pp. 30–32.
6. Susan Dimock, *Memoir of Susan Dimock* (Boston, 1875), p. 29.
7. Quoted in Putnam, *Life and Letters*, pp. 230, 232.
8. *Philadelphia Evening Bulletin*, 8 November 1869.
9. Diary of Sarah A. Hibbard, M.D., class of 1870, Archives and Special Collections on Women in Medicine, MS-54, Medical College of Pennsylvania, Philadelphia.
10. Northwestern University Medical School, Minutes of Faculty Meeting, 10 June 1870, Northwestern University Archives.
11. Chicago Medical Society, Minutes, October 1869, Chicago Historical Society.
12. *A Compendium of the Ninth Census (June 1, 1870)* (Washington: Government Printing Office, 1872), p. 606.

*1. Women and the Study of Medicine*

1. Mary A. E. Wager, "Women as Physicians," *Galaxy*, 1868, *6:* 781.

2. The six women who graduated from Western Reserve between 1852 and 1856, aside from Clark, were Emily Blackwell, Marie Zakrzewska, Sarah Chadwick, Cordelia Greene, and Elizabeth Griselle. Linda Goldstein, "Without Compromise of Delicate Feeling" (paper delivered at the sixtieth meeting of the American Association for the History of Medicine, May 1987, Philadelphia).

3. Thomas N. Bonner, *Medicine in Chicago, 1850–1950: A Chapter in the Social and Scientific Development of a City* (Madison, Wis.: American History Research Center, 1957), p. 61.

4. Wager, "Women as Physicians," p. 781.

5. Harriot K. Hunt, *Glances and Glimpses; or Fifty Years Social, Including Twenty Years Professional Life* (Boston: John P. Jewett, 1856), pp. 265–269; Ruth Caldwell, "The Pioneer Medical Woman," *Medical Woman's Journal*, 1930, *37:* 130.

6. Hunt, *Glances and Glimpses*, p. 270.

7. Marie Zakrzewska, "Fifty Years Ago—A Retrospect," *Women's Medical Journal*, 1893, *1:* 194.

8. Autobiography of Hannah Longshore, Archives and Special Collections on Women in Medicine, Medical College of Pennsylvania, MS-75, p. 3.

9. Sophia Jex-Blake, *Medical Women: A Thesis and a History* (Edinburgh: Oliphant, Anderson, & Ferrier, 1886), notes, p. 95; Louisa Garrett Anderson, *Elizabeth Garrett Anderson, 1836–1917* (London: Faber and Faber, [1939]), p. 286. I am indebted to Mary Ann C. Elston of University College London for explaining that the 1858 Medical Registration Act did not outlaw unregistered practice but made it very difficult for unregistered practitioners to find employment. Letter to author, 12 August 1988.

10. J. Steudel, "Heilkundige Frauen des Abendlandes," *Zentralblatt für Gynäkologie*, 1959, *81:* 285.

11. Kaethe Schirmacher, *The Modern Woman's Rights Movement* (New York: Macmillan, 1912), p. 160; Agnes Bluhm, "Die Entwicklung und der gegenwärtige Stand des medicinischen Frauenstudiums in den europäischen und aussereuropäischen Ländern," *Deutsche medizinische Wochenschrift*, 1895, *21:* 650.

12. Schirmacher, *Modern Woman's Rights Movement*, p. 160.

13. Elisabeth Burger, "Die Entwicklung des medizinischen Frauenstudiums" (dissertation, University of Marburg, 1947), p. 20.

14. Elizabeth Fee, "Science and the 'Woman Question': A Study of English Scientific Periodicals" (Ph.D. dissertation, Princeton University, 1978), p. 3.

15. Sara M. Evans, *Born for Liberty: A History of Women in America* (New York: Free Press, 1989), pp. 68–69.

16. See Carroll Smith-Rosenberg and Charles Rosenberg, "The Female Animal: Medical and Biological Views of Woman and Her Role in Nineteenth-

Century America," *Journal of American History,* 1973, 60: 332–356.

17. D. Hayes Agnew, *Introductory Lecture to the One Hundred and Fifth Course of Instruction in the Medical Department of the University of Pennsylvania* (Philadelphia: R. P. King's Son, 1870), p. 14.

18. *Boston Medical and Surgical Journal,* 1849, 40: 1.

19. Johanna Geyer-Kordesch, "Realisierung und Verlust 'weiblicher Identität' bei erfolgreicher Frauen: Die ersten Ärztinnengeneration und ihre Medizinkritik," in *Wie männlich ist die Wissenschaft?* ed. Karin Hausen and Helga Nowotny (Frankfurt am Main: Suhrkamp, 1986), pp. 214–215.

20. See the discussion of the educational opportunities for women in Onfel Thomas, *Frances Elizabeth Hoggan, 1843–1927* (privately printed, [1970]), p. 9.

21. Steudel, "Heilkundige Frauen des Abendlandes," p. 285.

22. Theodor L. W. von Bischoff, *Das Studium und die Ausübung der Medicin durch Frauen* (Munich: Literarisch-Artistische Anstalt, 1872), pp. 19–46.

23. Agnes C. Vietor, ed., *A Woman's Quest: The Life of Marie E. Zakrzewska, M.D.* (New York: D. Appleton, 1924), p. 140.

24. Jex-Blake, *Medical Women,* p. 72.

25. Jo Manton, *Elizabeth Garrett Anderson* (New York: E. P. Dutton, 1965), p. 73.

26. Mélanie Lipinska, *Histoire des femmes médecins depuis l'antiquité jusqu'à nos jours* (Paris: Librairie G. Jacques, 1900), p. 412.

27. Elizabeth Blackwell, *Pioneer Work in Opening the Medical Profession to Women* (London: Longman's, Green, 1895), p. 124.

28. Nancy A. Sahli, "Elizabeth Blackwell, M.D. (1821–1910): A Biography" (Ph.D. dissertation, University of Pennsylvania, 1974), p. 80.

29. Ruth Putnam, ed., *Life and Letters of Mary Putnam Jacobi* (New York: G. P. Putnam's Sons, 1925), p. 121.

30. Richard H. Shryock, "Women in American Medicine," *Journal of the American Medical Women's Association,* 1950, 5: 376.

31. Regina M. Morantz-Sanchez, *Sympathy and Science: Women Physicians in American Medicine* (New York: Oxford University Press, 1985), p. 99.

32. Putnam, *Life and Letters,* p. 67.

33. Vietor, *A Woman's Quest,* p. 256.

34. Ibid., pp. 178–181.

35. Blackwell, *Pioneer Work,* pp. 197–198.

36. Gulielma F. Alsop, *History of the Woman's Medical College, Philadelphia, Pennsylvania* (Philadelphia: J. B. Lippincott, 1950), p. 31. The college was called the Female Medical College of Pennsylvania until 1867.

37. Harold J. Abrahams, *Extinct Medical Schools of Nineteenth-Century Philadelphia* (Philadelphia: University of Pennsylvania Press, 1966), p. 550.

38. Esther P. Lovejoy, *Women Doctors of the World* (New York: Macmillan, 1957), pp. 8–18, 51.

39. Morantz-Sanchez, *Sympathy and Science,* p. 49.

40. Hunt, *Glances and Glimpses,* p. 359.

41. Frederick C. Waite, "Medical Education of Women in Cleveland," *Western*

*Reserve University Bulletin* no. 16, 15 September 1930, pp. 14–15, 20. The statements concerning Cincinnati, Cleveland, and San Francisco are based on this source.

42. Mary Putnam Jacobi, "Women in Medicine," in *What America Owes to Women*, ed. Lydia Hoyt Farmer (Buffalo: National Exposition Souvenir, 1893), p. 384.

43. I am indebted to Professor Atwater for sending me a copy of his paper "Women Who Became Doctors before the Civil War."

44. *A Compendium of the Ninth Census (June 1, 1870)* (Washington: Government Printing Office, 1872), pp. 493–504.

45. Mary Wright Pierson to correspondent, 11 December 1854, "Physicians, U.S." box, folder 35, Sophia Smith Collection, Smith College, Northampton, Massachusetts.

46. Morantz-Sanchez, *Sympathy and Science*, p. 69. See, too, the recent essay by Naomi Rogers in *Women, Health, and Medicine in America*, ed. Rima D. Apple (New York: Garland, 1990), pp. 281–310, which calls for a new approach to women sectarians, who "have been mostly left out of women's medical history" (p. 292).

47. Abrahams, *Extinct Medical Schools*, pp. 177–202.

48. Samuel Gregory, *Letter to Ladies, in Favor of Female Physicians for Their Own Sex* (Boston: Female Medical Education Society, 1850), p. 37.

49. Ibid.

50. *Boston Herald*, 10 September 1847.

51. Female Medical Education Society, Record Book, 13 July 1850, MS, Boston University Library, Boston.

52. Ibid., 23 November 1848.

53. See the *Announcement of a Course of Medical Lectures to Women in the City of Boston by the Faculty of the Female Medical College of Pennsylvania* (Boston, 1851) in the Archives and Special Collections on Women in Medicine at the Medical College of Pennsylvania (MCP). "It has been deemed advisable, for the present at least," reads the *Announcement* (p. 9), "for the Faculty of the Female Medical College of Pennsylvania, in conjunction with the New England Female Medical College, to give a full and thorough course of lectures in the city of Boston . . . during the ensuing spring."

54. Though sketchy, the *History of the New England Female Medical College, 1848–1874* (Boston: Boston University School of Medicine, 1950) by Frederick C. Waite is still the best account of the college. By Waite's count, 44 of the nongraduates eventually earned the medical degree at another college (pp. 85–89).

55. Alsop, *History of the Woman's Medical College*, p. 19. See, too, Clara Marshall, *The Woman's Medical College of Pennsylvania* (Philadelphia: P. Blakiston, 1897).

56. Minutes of the Board of Corporators, vol. 1: 1850–1856, 4 January 1850, Archives and Special Collections, MCP, A-1.

57. Thomas E. Longshore, History of the College, MS, Archives and Special Collections, MCP, C-4.

58. Cited by Martha Tracy in an unpublished address, "Five Pioneers," Archives

and Special Collections, MCP, C-4, p. 2.

59. Woman's Medical College of Pennsylvania, Faculty Minutes, 20 April 1852, Archives and Special Collections, MCP, C-4b.

60. Longshore, History of the College, p. 4.

61. *Olive Branch,* 17 January 1852, New England Female Medical College Scrapbook, Countway Library, Harvard Medical School.

62. Autobiography of Thomas Longshore, Archives and Special Collections, MCP, MS-75.

63. Pauline P. Foster, "Ann Preston, M.D. (1813–1872), A Biography: The Struggle to Obtain Training and Acceptance for Women Physicians in Mid-Nineteenth Century America" (Ph.D. dissertation, University of Pennsylvania, 1984), pp. 235–236.

64. Alsop, *History,* p. 91.

65. For the history of the Woman's Medical College of Baltimore, see Harold J. Abrahams, *The Extinct Medical Schools of Baltimore, Maryland* (Baltimore: Maryland Historical Society, 1969), pp. 71–131. This school will be considered more extensively in Chapter 7.

66. Vietor, *A Woman's Quest,* pp. 216–217.

67. Woman's Medical College of the New York Infirmary, *Final Catalogue,* p. 11.

68. Ibid., p. 12.

69. Mary Putnam Jacobi, "Woman in Medicine," in *Woman's Work in America,* ed. Annie Nathan Meyer (New York: Holt, 1891), p. 171; James R. Chadwick, *The Study and Practice of Medicine by Women* (New York: A. G. Barnes, 1879), p. 460.

70. Thomas N. Bonner, "Mary Harris Thompson," in *Notable American Women,* 3 vols., ed. Edward T. James and Janet W. James (Cambridge, Mass.: Belknap Press of Harvard University Press, 1971), 3: 454–455; Minutes of Faculty, Woman's Hospital Medical College of Chicago, 10 August 1870, Archives and Special Collections, MCP.

71. Helga M. Rudd, "The Women's [sic] Medical College of Chicago: Later Called the Northwestern University Woman's Medical College, 1870–1902," *Medical Woman's Journal,* 1946, 53: 42.

72. *Chicago Medical Examiner,* 1870, p. 586.

73. Bonner, *Medicine in Chicago,* pp. 61–62; Lovejoy, *Women Doctors,* pp. 92–93.

74. Vietor, *A Woman's Quest,* p. 414. See, too, Jacobi, "Woman in Medicine," p. 185.

75. "Women as Physicians," reprint from *Philadelphia Medical and Surgical Reports,* in "Women Physicians" collection, Countway Library, Harvard Medical School.

76. *Boston Medical and Surgical Journal,* 1853, 48: 66.

77. Zakrzewska, "Fifty Years Ago," p. 194.

78. Blackwell, *Pioneer Work,* p. 233.

79. Margaret Todd, *The Life of Sophia Jex-Blake* (London: Macmillan, 1918), p. 174.

80. Chadwick, *Study and Practice of Medicine,* p. 451.

81. Marshall, *Woman's Medical College of Pennsylvania*, pp. 11–12.
82. Hunt, *Glances and Glimpses*, pp. 271–272.
83. Vietor, *A Woman's Quest*, p. 277.
84. Jacobi, "Woman in Medicine," pp. 145–162.
85. Elizabeth Blackwell, *Address on the Medical Education of Women* (New York: Baptist and Taylor, 1864), p. 8.
86. *Report of the Commissioner of Education for the Year 1870* (Washington: Government Printing Office, 1875), p. 395.
87. Graham N. Fitch to John McLean, 29 January 1849, McLean Papers, John Crerar Library, Chicago.
88. Morantz-Sanchez, *Sympathy and Science*, p. 64.
89. Elizabeth and Emily Blackwell, *Medicine as a Profession for Women* (New York: W. H. Tinson, 1860), p. 19.
90. Blackwell, *Pioneer Work*, p. 238.
91. Vietor, *A Woman's Quest*, p. 400.
92. Todd, *Life of Jex-Blake*, pp. 190–192; Mary Roth Walsh, *"Doctors Wanted, No Women Need Apply": Sexual Barriers in the Medical Profession, 1835–1975* (New Haven: Yale University Press, 1977), pp. 166–168.
93. Franziska Tiburtius, "The Development of the Study of Medicine for Women in Germany, and Present Status," *Canadian Practitioner and Review*, 1909, *34:* 498.
94. Virginia G. Drachman, *Hospital with a Heart: Women Doctors and the Paradox of Separatism at the New England Hospital, 1862–1969* (Ithaca: Cornell University Press, 1984), pp. 66–67.
95. History of the New England Women's Medical Society, MS, Margaret Noyes Kleinert Papers, Schlesinger Library, Radcliffe College, Cambridge, Massachusetts.
96. Caroline H. Dall, ed., *A Practical Illustration of "Woman's Right to Labor" or A Letter from Marie E. Zakrzewska, M.D., Late of Berlin, Prussia* (Boston: Walker, Wise and Co., 1860), p. 130.
97. Sahli, "Elizabeth Blackwell," pp. 141–142.
98. Putnam, *Life and Letters*, pp. 239–240.
99. Dimock, *Memoir*, p. 60.
100. Lovejoy, *Women Doctors*, p. 99.
101. Ibid., pp. 49, 52.
102. Untitled manuscript by Frederick C. Waite, "Schools and Societies," folder 74, Sophia Smith Collection, Smith College.
103. Morantz-Sanchez, *Sympathy and Science*, p. 167.
104. Vietor, *A Woman's Quest*, pp. 490, 496–497.
105. Ibid., p. 490.
106. Chadwick, *Study and Practice of Medicine by Women*, p. 460.
107. Lovejoy, *Women Doctors*, p. 92.
108. Martin Kaufman, Stuart Galishoff, and Todd L. Savitt, eds., *Dictionary of American Medical Biography*, 2 vols. (Westport, Conn.: Greenwood Press, 1984). To be listed, a physician must have died before 31 December 1976. If only regular physicians are counted and not sectarians, the proportion of women going abroad is even higher.

109. Bonner, *American Doctors and German Universities*, pp. 28–29.
110. Walsh, "Doctors Wanted," table 5, p. 186. The eleven were Elizabeth Blackwell, the six graduates of the Western Reserve Medical College (note 2), Mary Thompson, Mary Putnam, Susan Dimock, and Martha A. Rogers. The last graduated from the Geneva Medical College in 1865 before the school was moved to Syracuse. See Waite, "The Medical Education of Women in Cleveland," p. 6.
111. Vietor, *A Woman's Quest*, pp. 358–359.
112. See Dorothy G. McGuigan, *A Dangerous Experiment: 100 Years of Women at the University of Michigan* (Ann Arbor: Center for Continuing Education of Women, 1970), pp. 35–38.
113. Quoted in Vietor, *A Woman's Quest*, pp. 342–343.
114. "Women Physicians," *Macmillan's Magazine*, September 1868, p. 370.
115. Wilhelm von Zehender, *Ueber den Beruf der Frauen zum Studium und zur praktischen Ausbildung der Heilwissenschaft* (Rostock: Stiller'sche Hof- und Universitätsbuchhandlung, 1875), pp. 18–19.

## 2. Zurich and Paris

1. Gordon A. Craig, *The Triumph of Liberalism: Zürich in the Golden Age, 1830–1869* (New York: Scribner's, 1988), p. x.
2. Ibid., p. 151.
3. Susanna Woodtli, *Gleichberechtigung: Der Kampf um die politischen Rechte der Frau in der Schweiz*, rev. ed. (Frauenfeld: Huber, 1983), pp. 75–76.
4. The correspondence concerning Kniaszhnina is found in the Staatsarchiv in Zurich, section on Frauenstudium 1864–1879, general correspondence file in box 49416, especially the letters of 28 November 1864 and 15 January 1865.
5. The best source of general information about Zurich in English is Craig, *Triumph of Liberalism*.
6. Elaine Schwöbel-Schrafl, *Was verdankt die medizinische Fakultät Zürich ihren ausländischen Dozenten? 1833 bis 1863* (Zurich: Juris Druck & Verlag, 1985), p. 16.
7. Ibid., p. 31.
8. Ibid., p. 47.
9. Ernst Gagliardi, Hans Nabholz, and Jean Strohl, *Die Universität Zürich, 1833–1933: Festschrift zur Jahrhundertfeier* (Zurich: Verlag der Erziehungsdirektion, 1938), p. 552.
10. Barbara A. Engel, "Women Medical Students in Russia, 1872–1882: Reformers or Rebels?" *Journal of Social History*, 1978, *12:* 394–397; Christine Johanson, "Autocratic Politics, Public Opinion, and Women's Medical Education during the Reign of Alexander II, 1855–1881," *Slavic Review*, 1979, *38:* 426–431; and Cynthia H. Whittaker, "The Women's Movement during the Reign of Alexander II: A Case Study in Russian Liberalism," *Journal of Modern History*, 1976, *48:* 40–42.
11. J. M. Meijer, *Knowledge and Revolution: The Russian Colony in Zurich (1870–1873)* (Assen, Netherlands: Van Gorcum, 1955), pp. 23–24; Hanny Rohner,

*Die ersten 30 Jahre des medizinischen Frauenstudiums an der Universität Zürich, 1867–1897* (Zurich: Juris Druck & Verlag, 1972), p. 17.

12. Protokoll der medizinischen Fakultät Zürich, 1864–1890, minutes of 29 January 1867, University of Zurich Archives; Victor Böhmert, *Das Studieren der Frauen mit besonderer Rücksicht auf das Studium der Medicin* (Leipzig: Otto Wigand, 1872), pp. 1–5; Rohner, *Die ersten 30 Jahre*, p. 12; Woodtli, *Gleichberechtigung*, p. 78.

13. Gagliardi et al., *Die Universität Zürich*, pp. 89–91; Ludimar Hermann, *Erinnerungen* (Berlin: privately printed, 1915), p. 82; Franziska Tiburtius, *Erinnerungen einer Achtzigjährigen*, 3rd ed. (Berlin: C. A. Schwetschke, 1929), pp. 159–162.

14. See biography of Böhmert in *Neue Deutsche Biographie, 2:* 394–395 and his autobiography, *Rückblicke und Ausblicke eines Siebzigers* (Dresden: O. V. Böhmert, 1900).

15. Schweizerischer Verband der Akademikerinnen, *Das Frauenstudium an den Schweizer Hochschulen* (Zurich: Rascher & Cie, 1928), p. 59.

16. August Forel, *Rückblick auf mein Leben* (Zurich: Europa-Verlag, 1934), p. 45.

17. Arthur Kirchoff, *Die akademische Frau: Gutachten hervorragender Universitätsprofessoren, Frauenlehrer und Schriftsteller über die Befähigung der Frau zum wissenschaftlichen Studium und Berufe* (Berlin: Hugo Steinitz, 1897), p. 71.

18. V. A. Bazanov, "Nadezhda Suslova—pervaii russkaii zhenschina-vrach," *Fel'dsher i akusherka* (Moscow), 1963, 9: 53.

19. For Erismann, see Hanspeter Wick, *Friedrich Huldreich Erismann (1842–1915): Russischer Hygieniker—Zürcher Stadtrat* (Zurich: Zürcher Medizingeschichtliche Abhandlungen, n.s. 82, 1970).

20. The description of the examination is from Victor Böhmert, *Das Studium der Frauen an der Universität Zürich* (Zurich, 1870), p. 2. The Rose quotation is from a Russian source cited in Jeanette Tuve, *The First Russian Women Physicians* (Newtonville, Mass.: Oriental Research Partners, 1984), p. 21.

21. Monika Bankowski-Züllig, "Zürich—das russische Mekka," in *Ebenso neu als kühn: 120 Jahre Frauenstudium an der Universität Zürich* (Zurich: Verein Feministische Wissenschaft Schweiz, 1988), p. 127.

22. For Morgan, see Onfel Thomas, *Frances Elizabeth Hoggan, 1843–1927* (privately printed, [1970]), pp. 7–11.

23. Rohner, *Die ersten 30 Jahre*, pp. 28–29.

24. Forel to his mother, 19 June 1869, Medizinhistorisches Institut, University of Zurich.

25. Thomas, *Frances Elizabeth Hoggan*, p. 12.

26. August Forel, *Out of My Life and Work* (New York: Norton, 1937), p. 56.

27. August Forel, *Briefe—Correspondance, 1864–1927,* ed. Hans H. Walser (Bern, 1968), p. 63.

28. The following account of the examination is from Victor Böhmert, *Die zweite Doctorpromotion einer Dame in Zürich* (Zurich, 1870), pp. 1–7.

29. Forel, *Rückblick auf mein Leben*, pp. 45–46.

30. Ibid., p. 46.

31. *Medical Women's Federation Newsletter*, 1925, pp. 58–59. I am indebted to Mary Ann Elston of University College, London, for a copy of this brief obituary.

32. Rohner, *Die ersten 30 Jahre*, p. 29; Schweizerischer Verband, *Das Frauenstudium*, p. 31.

33. Bankowski-Züllig, "Zürich—das russische Mekka," p. 129.

34. Forel to mother, 19 June 1869, Medizinhistorisches Institut, Zurich.

35. Johanna Siebel, *Das Leben von Frau Dr. Marie Heim-Vögtlin 1845–1916* (Zurich: Rascher & Cie, 1928), p. 64.

36. Edmund Rose, *Der Zürcher Hülfszug zum Schlachtfeld bei Belfort* (Zurich: Cäsar Schmidt, 1871), p. 17.

37. Susan Dimock, *Memoir of Susan Dimock* (Boston, 1875), pp. 5–13.

38. Ibid., pp. 13–14.

39. Obituary of Susan Dimock, *Medical Record*, 15 May 1875, p. 357.

40. Siebel, *Das Leben von Frau Dr. Heim-Vögtlin*, pp. 59–60.

41. Ibid. The following account of Vögtlin's life is taken from the Siebel biography.

42. Ibid., p. 46.

43. Rohner, *Die ersten 30 Jahre*, p. 44.

44. Dimock, *Memoir*, pp. 16–17.

45. Dimock to Samuel Cabot, 25 October 1868, Sophia Smith Collection, Smith College, Northampton, Massachusetts.

46. Dimock, *Memoir*, p. 19.

47. Siebel, *Das Leben von Frau Dr. Heim-Vögtlin*, pp. 59–60.

48. Ibid., p. 60.

49. Böhmert, *Das Studium der Frauen* (1872), p. 24.

50. Rohner, *Die ersten 30 Jahre*, pp. 44–45.

51. The best contemporary account of these developments is another of Victor Böhmert's articles, *Das Frauenstudium nach den Erfahrungen an der Züricher Universität* (Leipzig, 1874). For a list of the names and addresses of the Russian women in Zurich, see the careful compilation by Monika Bankowski-Züllig in *Ebenso neu als kühn*, pp. 140–145.

52. Monika Bankowski-Züllig, "Russische Studierende in der Schweiz," in *Schweiz-Russland: Begleitband zur Ausstellung der Präsidialabteilung der Stadt Zürich*, ed. Werner G. Zimmermann (Zurich: Strauhof Zürich, 1989), pp. 81–82. See, too, idem, "Russischer Alltag im Plattenquartier," *Uni Zürich*, April 1986, pp. 10–12.

53. Tiburtius, *Erinnerungen*, pp. 124–130, 152–154; Johannes Scherr, *Die Nihilisten* (Leipzig: Otto Wigand, 1885), p. 112; Hans Erb, *Geschichte der Studentenschaft an der Universität Zürich, 1833–1936* (Zurich: Werder & Co., 1937), pp. 70–72.

54. Dimock to Cabot, 9 October 1873, Sophia Smith Collection, Smith College.

55. Tiburtius, *Erinnerungen*, pp. 128, 156.

56. Katharina Gundling, "Weibliche Studenten in Zürich," *Der Bazar* [Berlin], 21 August 1871, 32: 262.

57. Engel, "Women Medical Students in Russia," pp. 404–405. Richard Stites estimates that "less than a quarter" of the women students were radicals and that "it is clear that a large majority of the female medical students were there for serious study alone." Stites, *The Women's Liberation Movement in Russia: Feminism, Nihilism, and Bolshevism, 1860–1930* (Princeton: Princeton University Press, 1978), p. 84.
58. Johanson, "Autocratic Politics," p. 434.
59. Quoted in Meijer, *Knowledge and Revolution,* p. 48.
60. Böhmert, *Das Studieren der Frauen* (1872), p. 21.
61. The text of the Russian ban on women studying in Zurich and the students' response is found in Anon., *Die Verläumdung der in Zürich studierenden russischen Frauen durch die russische Regierung* (Zurich: Genossenschafts-Buchdruckerei, [1873]), pp. 3–11. See, too, Tuve, *First Russian Women Physicians,* p. 25.
62. H. Henke, *Statistik der Universität Zürich in den ersten fünfzig Jahren ihres Bestehens von Ostern 1833 bis Ostern 1883* (Zurich: Zürcher und Furrer, 1883), p. 52.
63. Daniela Neumann, *Studentinnen aus dem Russischen Reich in der Schweiz (1867–1914)* (Zurich: Hans Rohr, 1987), pp. 124–125; Bankowski-Züllig, "Zürich—das russische Mekka," p. 128. Neumann gives a range of 18 to 30 percent who finished their degrees, while Bankowski estimates that one-fifth did. My own estimate is nearer 25 percent.
64. Neumann, *Studentinnen,* pp. 128–129.
65. Rohner, *Die ersten 30 Jahre,* p. 14.
66. Ibid.
67. Böhmert, *Das Studieren der Frauen* (1872), p. 22.
68. Ibid., p. 44.
69. Böhmert, *Das Studium der Frauen* (1870), pp. 6–7.
70. Emilie Benz, ed., *Die Frauenbewegung in der Schweiz* (Zurich: Th. Schröter, 1902), p. 55.
71. Ludimar Hermann, *Das Frauenstudium und die Interessen der Hochschule Zürich* (Zurich, 1872), pp. 5–7.
72. Meijer, *Knowledge and Revolution,* pp. 145–156.
73. Tuve, *The First Russian Women Physicians,* pp. 34–43.
74. Meijer, *Knowledge and Revolution,* p. 146.
75. Caroline Schultze, *La femme-médecin au XIXᵉ siècle* (Paris: Librairie Ollier-Henry, 1888), table, p. 15.
76. Roland Nahon, "Contribution à l'étude de l'accession des femmes à la carrière médicale à la fin du XIXᵉ siècle" (doctoral thesis, University of Paris Val de Marne, Faculté de Médecine, 1978), p. 10.
77. The text of the Duruy proposal is in "Une conquête du feminisme sous le Second Empire: Fondation d'une école pour l'instruction médicale des femmes," *Bulletin de l'enseignement public au Maroc,* 1954, *229:* 51–61. The proposal was never revived after the collapse of the Second Empire.
78. Women's Medical Association of New York City, *Mary Putnam Jacobi, M.D.: A Pathfinder in Medicine* (New York: G. P. Putnam's Sons, 1925), p. xiii.

79. Ruth Putnam, ed., *Life and Letters of Mary Putnam Jacobi* (New York: G. P. Putnam's Sons, 1925), p. 287.

80. Reprinted in Putnam, *Life and Letters,* p. 290. Putnam was English by birth, having been born when her parents were abroad.

81. Jo Manton, *Elizabeth Garrett Anderson* (New York: E. P. Dutton, 1965), p. 53. This and the following paragraph are based on the Manton book and Louisa Garrett Anderson, *Elizabeth Garrett Anderson, 1836–1917* (London: Faber and Faber, 1939).

82. Manton, *Elizabeth Garrett Anderson,* p. 109.

83. Gilbert Percebois, "Les femmes à la conquête de la médecine," *Annales médicales de Nancy,* 1977, p. 1262.

84. *The Lancet,* 18 June 1870.

85. Mélanie Lipinska, *Histoire des femmes médecins* (Paris: Librairie G. Jacques, 1900), p. 418.

86. Percebois, "Les femmes à la conquête," p. 1262.

87. H. Montanier, "La femme médecin," *Gazette des hôpitaux,* 1868, *34:* pp. 1–2. Some of the early debate is found in Augustine Girault (pseud. A. Gaël), *La femme médecin: sa raison d'être au point de vue du droit, de la moralité et de l'humanité* (Paris: E. Dentu, 1868).

88. G.R. in *L'Union médicale,* 1875, *3:* 26–27.

89. E.T. in *Le Progrès médical,* 29 May 1875.

90. E. Beaugrand in *Dictionnaire encyclopédique des sciences médicales,* 18th ed., 1874, p. 605.

91. Ibid., p. 606.

92. Across the matriculation record of Mary Putnam is scrawled: "Seize [credits]—allouées pour équivalence de diplôm de docteur en médecine de Philadelphia et de pharmacien de New York (Etats Unis)—l'action du 4 Juin 1868." Mary Putnam file, matriculation records of Faculté de Médecine de Paris, Archives Nationales, Paris.

93. George Weisz, *The Emergence of Modern Universities in France, 1863–1914* (Princeton: Princeton University Press, 1983), pp. 243–247. Even in Switzerland, because of the strict separation of the sexes, women were forced to find alternatives to public secondary schools. It was not until 1891 that women were admitted to classes in the Swiss *Gymnasium.* Johannes Steudel, "Medical Women of the Occident," *Journal of the American Medical Women's Association,* 1962, *17:* 53.

94. The Zurich figures are found in the matriculation books of the University of Zurich, 1833–1933, in the Staatsarchiv, Zurich; the Bern numbers are in Marianne Progin and Werner Seitz, "Das Frauenstudium an der Universitaet Bern" (paper for Historisches Seminar, University of Bern, September 1980); and the early Paris enrollments are listed in Lipinska, *Histoire des femmes médecins,* p. 416.

95. Women's Medical Association, *Mary Putnam Jacobi,* p. xiv.

96. Vietor, *A Woman's Quest,* p. 359.

97. Lovejoy, *Women Doctors of the World,* p. 165.

98. Ibid., pp. 176–206.

99. Johanson, "Autocratic Politics," p. 435.

100. Tiburtius, "Development of the Study of Medicine for Women in Germany," p. 492.

101. Jex-Blake, *Medical Women*, appendix, p. 84.

102. Robert W. Johnson, "Impressions of Vienna as a Medical School," *Philadelphia Medical Times*, 1880, *11:* 138.

## 3. The Great Migration

1. Mary Putnam Jacobi, "Women in Medicine," in *What America Owes to Women*, ed. Lydia Hoyt Farmer (Buffalo: National Exposition Souvenir, 1893), p. 387. For Dimock, see the remarkable tributes in Susan Dimock, *Memoir* (Boston, 1875).

2. Jo Manton, *Elizabeth Garrett Anderson* (New York: E. P. Dutton, 1965), pp. 240–268.

3. Agnes Bluhm, "Die Entwicklung und der gegenwärtige Stand des medicinischen Frauenstudiums in den europäischen und aussereuropäischen Ländern," *Deutsche medizinische Wochenschrift*, 1895, *21:* 650.

4. Jeanette E. Tuve, *The First Russian Women Physicians* (Newtonville, Mass.: Oriental Research Partners, 1984), pp. 23–27.

5. Ibid., pp. 17, 27.

6. Monika Bankowski-Züllig, "Zürich—das russische Mekka," in *Ebenso neu als kühn: 120 Jahre Frauenstudium an der Universität Zürich* (Zurich: Verein Feministische Wissenschaft Schweiz, 1988), pp. 132–133.

7. See Zbigniew Filar, *Anna Tomaszewicz Dobrska: A Leaf from Polish Medical History* (Warsaw: Polish Society of the History of Medicine, 1959).

8. Barbara A. Engel and Clifford N. Rosenthal, eds., *Five Sisters: Women against the Tsar* (Boston: Allen & Unwin, 1987), p. 146.

9. Schweizerischer Verband der Akademikerinnen, *Das Frauenstudium an den Schweizer Hochschulen* (Zurich: Rascher & Cie, 1928), pp. 1–2.

10. Helene Lange, *Higher Education of Women in Europe*, trans. L. R. Klemm (New York: D. Appleton, 1890), p. xxi.

11. Ibid., pp. xxiv, xxv.

12. *Compendium of the Tenth Census (June 1, 1880)*, 2 parts (Washington: Government Printing Office, 1883), *2:* 1368.

13. Franziska Tiburtius, "The Development of the Study of Medicine for Women in Germany, and Present Status," *Canadian Practitioner and Review*, 1909, *34:* 492.

14. Women's Medical Association of New York City, ed., *Mary Putnam Jacobi, M.D.: A Pathfinder in Medicine* (New York: G. P. Putnam's Sons, 1925), p. 355.

15. Emily F. Pope, Emma L. McCall, and C. Augusta Pope, *The Practice of Medicine by Women in the United States* (Boston: Wright & Potter, 1881), p. 12.

16. James R. Chadwick, *The Study and Practice of Medicine by Women* (New York: A. S. Barnes, 1879), p. 471.

17. James J. Putnam, "Women at Zurich," *Boston Medical and Surgical Journal,* 1879, *101:* 567.

18. *Boston Medical and Surgical Journal,* 1879, *101:* 460.

19. Ibid., 567.

20. Lawson Tait, "The Medical Education of Women," *Birmingham Medical Review,* 1874, pp. 81–94. Tait visited the surgical clinic of Edmund Rose in Zurich, the anatomy class of Hermann Meyer, and the medical clinic of Anton Biermer, and came away impressed with the ability of the women students and the lack of discomfort on the part of professors and students.

21. Frances Elizabeth [Morgan] Hoggan, "Women in Medicine," in *The Woman Question in Europe,* ed. Theodore Stanton (New York: G. P. Putnam's Sons, 1884), pp. 82–84.

22. J. Steudel, "Medical Women of the Occident," *Journal of the American Medical Women's Association,* 1962, *17:* 52.

23. Lange, *Higher Education of Women,* p. 1.

24. Arthur Kirchoff, *Die akademische Frau: Gutachten hervorragender Universitätsprofessoren, Frauenlehrer und Schriftsteller über die Befähigung der Frau zum wissenschaftlichen Studium und Berufe* (Berlin: Hugo Steinitz, 1897), table, p. 362; Barbara Engel, "Women Medical Students in Russia, 1872–1882: Reformers or Rebels?" *Journal of Social History,* 1978, *12:* 407.

25. The estimates are based on the following sources: Matrikel der Universität Zürich, 1833–1933, Staatsarchiv, Zurich; Barbara Bachmann and Elke Bradenahl, "Medizinstudium von Frauen in Bern, 1871–1914" (dissertation, University of Bern, 1990), pp. 17–18; the tables in Marianne Progin and Werner Seitz, "Das Frauenstudium an der Universitaet Bern" (paper for Historisches Seminar, University of Bern, September 1980); *Bulletin administratif du Ministère de l'Instruction Publique,* Paris, 1899–1914; Université de Genève, *Historique des Facultés, 1896–1914* (Geneva: Georg & Co., Libraires de l'Université, 1914), table, p. 285; Charles Borgeaud, ed., *Histoire de l'Université de Genève,* 4 vols. (Geneva: Georg & Co., Libraires de l'Université, 1934), 3 (annexes): 290; Université de Lausanne, *Cinquantenaire de la Faculté de Médecine de Lausanne, 1890–1940* (Lausanne: F. Roth & Co. [1940]); and Eidgenössisches Statistisches Amt, *Schweizerische Hochschulstatistik, 1890–1935* (Bern, 1935).

26. Hanny Rohner, *Die ersten 30 Jahre des medizinischen Frauenstudiums an der Universität Zurich, 1867–1897* (Zurich: Juris Druck & Verlag, 1972), p. 33.

27. Agnes C. Vietor, ed., *A Woman's Quest: The Life of Marie E. Zakrzewska, M.D.* (New York: D. Appleton, 1924), p. 383.

28. Pietro Scandola, *Hochschulgeschichte Berns, 1528–1984* (Bern: Universität Bern, 1984), p. 500.

29. Progin and Seitz, "Das Frauenstudium an der Universitaet Bern," pp. 13–14; Bachmann and Bradenahl, *Medizinstudium von Frauen,* table 4.1, p. 18.

30. Schweizerischer Verband, *Das Frauenstudium,* p. 64.

31. H. von Scheel, *Frauenfrage und Frauenstudium: Rectoratsrede gehalten am Stiftungstage der Hochschule zu Bern* (Jena: Druck der Friedrich Mauke'schen Officin, 1873), p. 1.

32. Ibid., pp. 4, 6–8, 13–14.
33. Bachmann and Bradenahl, *Medizinstudium von Frauen,* p. 18.
34. Franziska Tiburtius, *Erinnerungen einer Achtzigjährigen,* 3rd ed. (Berlin: C. A. Schwetschke, 1929), pp. 155–156; Rohner, *Die ersten 30 Jahre,* p. 23. Berlinerblau changed her name to Berlin in the United States.
35. Jex-Blake, *Medical Women,* appendix, p. 99.
36. Ibid., p. 55.
37. Information supplied by Professor E. Hintzsche of the Bern School of Medicine.
38. Progin and Seitz, "Das Frauenstudium an der Universitaet Bern," p. 17.
39. Schweizerischer Verband, *Das Frauenstudium,* p. 101.
40. Progin and Seitz, "Das Frauenstudium an der Universitaet Bern," p. 47.
41. Daniela Neumann, *Studentinnen aus dem Russischen Reich in der Schweiz (1867–1914)* (Zurich: Hans Rohr, 1987), p. 82.
42. M. Cramer and J. Starobinski, eds., *Centenaire de la Faculté de Médecine de l'Université de Genève: Documents* (Geneva: Editions Médecine et Hygiène, 1978), pp. 23, 37.
43. L. Mysyrowicz, "Université et révolution: Les étudiants d'Europe Orientale à Genève au temps de Plékhanov et de Lénine," *Revue Suisse d'Histoire,* 1975, *25:* 515–516.
44. Borgeaud, *Histoire de l'Université de Genève,* 3: 289.
45. Marie Goegg, "Switzerland," in *The Woman Question in Europe,* ed. Theodore Stanton (New York: G. P. Putnam's Sons, 1884), p. 387.
46. Ladislas Mysyrowicz, "Les étudiants 'orientaux' en médecine à Genève," *Gesnerus,* 1977, *34:* 209.
47. Université de Genève, *Historique des Facultés,* pp. 277–283.
48. Mysyrowicz, "Les étudiants 'orientaux,' " pp. 208–209.
49. Chaim Weizmann, *Trial and Error: The Autobiography of Chaim Weizmann* (New York: Harper, 1949), p. 71.
50. Mysyrowicz, "Université et révolution," p. 523.
51. Ibid.
52. Mysyrowicz, "Les étudiants 'orientaux,' " p. 210.
53. Mysyrowicz, "Université et révolution," pp. 527–528.
54. Université de Lausanne, *Cinquantenaire de la Faculté de Médecine de Lausanne, 1890–1940* (Lausanne: F. Roth & Co., [1940]), pp. 146–147.
55. Schweizerischer Verband, *Das Frauenstudium,* pp. 176, 188.
56. Ibid., p. 189.
57. The university rector at Basel, an obstetrician, in 1892 described the study of medicine by women as "always a certain exception" by persons destined to treat only women and children. They were subject to nerve and blood vessel "disturbances . . . that quite frequently approach the border of the pathological." H. Fehling, *Die Bestimmung der Frau,* pp. 16, 27. Professor Gustav von Bunge, in contrast, was the only member of the medical faculty to support the education of women. He wrote his stepmother in 1894 that the strict insistence by his colleagues on a Swiss diploma was "to keep away the Russian nihilists who were loathed by the proper citizens of

Basel." Marie-Louise Portmann, "Neue Aspekte zur Biographie des Basler Biochemikers Gustav von Bunge (1844–1920) aus seinem handschriftlichen Nachlass," *Gesnerus*, 1974, *31:* 44.

58. Eidgenössisches Statistisches Amt, *Schweizerische Hochschulstatistik*, p. 53.
59. A total of 56 American women registered in medicine at Zurich alone by 1900. Matrikel der Universität Zürich, 1833–1933, Staatsarchiv Zurich.
60. "American Women Students at Zurich University," *Woman's Medical Journal*, 1897, *6:* 303–304.
61. "Les étudiantes," *La France médicale*, 14 April 1883, p. 526.
62. Caroline Schultze, *La femme-médecin au XIXᵉ siècle* (Paris: Librairie Ollier-Henry, 1888), p. 16.
63. *Bulletin administratif du ministère de l'instruction publique*, no. 67, Jan.–June 1900, pp. 326–327.
64. Françoise Leguay and Claude Barbizet, *Blanche Edwards-Pilliet: Femme et médecin, 1858–1941* (Le Mans: Editions Cénomane, 1988), p. 40.
65. Constance Joël, *Les filles d'Esculape: Les femmes à la conquête du pouvoir médical* (Paris: Robert Laffont, 1988), p. 119.
66. Richard Satran, "Augusta Déjerine-Klumpke: First Woman Intern in Paris Hospitals," *Annals of Internal Medicine*, 1974, *80:* 262.
67. Roland Nahon, "Contribution à l'étude de l'accession des femmes à la carrière médicale à la fin du XIXᵉ siècle" (doctoral thesis, Université Paris Val de Marne, 1978), p. 13.
68. Satran, "Augusta Déjerine-Klumpke," p. 261. See, too, André-Thomas, "Augusta Déjerine-Klumpke, 1859–1927," *L'Encéphale*, February 1928, pp. 75–88, and "Madame Déjerine-Klumpke (1859–1927)," *La Presse médicale*, 14 November 1959.
69. Leguay and Barbizet, *Blanche Edwards-Pilliet*, p. 33.
70. Joël, *Les filles d'Esculape*, pp. 120–121.
71. Satran, "Augusta Déjerine-Klumpke," pp. 262–263.
72. *La France Médicale*, 1884, *31:* 1276, 1622.
73. *Revue Scientifique*, 1884, *34:* 538.
74. Paul Bert, "Les femmes et l'internat des hôpitaux," *Le Voltaire*, 29 September 1884.
75. Joël, *Les filles d'Esculape*, p. 121.
76. Quoted in Satran, "Augusta Déjerine-Klumpke," p. 263.
77. André-Thomas, "Augusta Déjerine-Klumpke," pp. 82–87.
78. Leguay and Barbizet, *Blanche Edwards-Pilliet*, p. 48.
79. G. Lhermitte, "Un Cinquantenaire," *Le droit des femmes*, February 1939, p. 20.
80. Leguay and Barbizet, *Blanche Edwards-Pilliet*, p. 48.
81. For Montpellier, see Claude Romieu, "Agnes McLaren, première femme docteur en médecine de la Faculté de Montpellier," *Monspeliensis Hippocrates*, 1966, *31:* 21–28.
82. Helene Lange, *Frauenbildung* (Berlin: L. Dehmigke, 1889), p. 75.
83. "Women Medical Students in Paris," *Woman's Medical Journal*, 1897, *6:* 239.

84. Mélanie Lipinska, *Histoire des femmes médecins* (Paris: G. Jacques, 1900), p. 530.

85. Ibid., p. 526.

86. See the list of all women doctorates in medicine in Haryett Fontanges, *Les femmes docteurs en médecine dans tous les pays*, 3rd ed. (Paris: Alliance Coopérative du Livre, 1901), pp. 77–104.

87. Schultze, *La femme médecin au XIXᵉ siècle*, p. 16.

88. Regina M. Morantz-Sanchez, *Sympathy and Science: Women Physicians in American Medicine* (New York: Oxford University Press, 1985), table 9-2, p. 245.

89. Elisabeth Burger, "Die Entwicklung des medizinischen Frauenstudiums" (doctoral dissertation, University of Marburg, 1947), p. 53.

90. Neumann, *Studentinnen aus dem Russischen Reich*, p. 205.

91. General Circular, Johns Hopkins University School of Medicine, "Schools and Societies" box, folder 68, Sophia Smith Collection, Smith College, Northampton, Massachusetts.

92. Natalia Oettli-Kirpichnikova, unpublished memoirs, pp. 208–209, cited in Neumann, *Studentinnen aus dem Russischen Reich*, p. 48.

93. Eidgenössisches Statistisches Amt, *Schweizerische Hochschulstatistik 1890–1935*, tables, pp. 54–55.

94. *Bulletin administratif du Ministère de l'instruction publique, 1900–1901*, pp. 236–237; *1905–1906*, pp. 470–471.

95. Ibid., *1913–1914*, pp. 270–271; Eidgenössisches Statistisches Amt, *Schweizerische Hochschulstatistik*, p. 54.

96. Progin and Seitz, "Das Frauenstudium an der Universitaet Bern," p. 20.

97. Schweizerischer Verband der Akademikerinnen, *Das Frauenstudium*, pp. 139–140; Mysyrowicz, "Les étudiants 'orientaux,' " pp. 209–210.

98. Ernst Gagliardi, Hans Nabholz, and Jean Strohl, *Die Universität Zürich 1833–1933: Festschrift zur Jahrhundertfeier* (Zurich: Erziehungsdirektion, 1938).

99. *La Semaine médicale*, 1914, *34*: C11. The data given in this publication cover all foreign medical students from 1896 to 1914. See, too, George Weisz, *The Emergence of Modern Universities in France, 1863–1914* (Princeton: Princeton University Press, 1983), table 7.11, p. 262. Weisz's figures show the following breakdown of foreign medical students, men as well as women, in 1914: Russian Empire, 62 percent; Balkans, 12 percent; Ottoman Empire and Middle East, 7 percent; Latin America and Caribbean, 5 percent; Northern and Central Europe, 5 percent; Southern Europe, 5 percent; Africa, 2 percent; Far East, 2 percent; United States and Canada, 1 percent.

100. George F. Jewsbury, "Russian Students in Nancy, France: 1905–1914. A Case Study," *Jahrbücher für Geschichte Osteuropas*, 1975, *23*: 227.

101. Mysyrowicz, "Université et révolution," pp. 528–529.

102. Dean to Regierungsrat Dr. Gobat, [1905], Staatsarchiv Bern, Mappe der medizinischen Fakultät.

103. J. Saurer and G. Beran, "Ausländische Studierende an der Universität Bern, 1834–1979" (paper for Historisches Seminar, University of Bern, [1980]), pp. 11–12.

104. Alfred E. Senn, *The Russian Revolution in Switzerland, 1914–1917* (Madison: University of Wisconsin Press, 1971), p. 7.
105. Alumnae files, Archives and Special Collections on Women in Medicine, Medical College of Pennsylvania; Catharine Macfarlane, "The Woman's Medical College of Pennsylvania," *Transactions and Studies of the College of Physicians and Surgeons of Philadelphia*, 1965, *33:* 39–42.
106. Nancy M. Frieden, *Russian Physicians in an Era of Reform and Revolution, 1856–1905* (Princeton: Princeton University Press, 1981), appendix IA, p. 323.
107. August Forel, *Rückblick auf mein Leben* (Zurich, 1934), p. 7.
108. University of Zurich Archives, Protokoll der medizinischen Fakultät Zürich, 1890–1912, meeting of 23 May 1890, p. 3.
109. Helen D. Webster, "Our Debt to Zurich," in *The World's Congress of Representative Women*, ed. May Wright Sewall (New York: Rand McNally, 1894), pp. 694–695.
110. Marianne Weber, "Vom Typenwandel der studierenden Frau," in *Frauenfragen und Frauengedanken: Gesammelte Aufsätze* (Tübingen: J. C. B. Mohr, 1919), pp. 179–194. The essay was written in 1917.

## 4. Women, Medicine, and Revolution in Russia

1. Barbara A. Engel and Clifford N. Rosenthal, eds., *Five Sisters: Women against the Tsar* (Boston: Allen & Unwin, 1987), p. xv.
2. See the discussion of the reasons for Russian women's greater zeal in Ruth A. Dudgeon, "Women and Higher Education in Russia, 1855–1905" (Ph.D. dissertation, George Washington University, 1975), pp. 388–390.
3. Nearly 1,700 Russians, the majority of them men, were studying medicine in Germany in 1912. *Münchener medizinische Wochenschrift*, 1913, *60:* 221. For Russian women in Germany, see Claudie Weill, "Les étudiants russes en Allemagne, 1900–1914," *Cahiers du monde russe et soviétique*, 1979, *20:* 214, and Elisabeth Burger, "Die Entwicklung des medizinischen Frauenstudiums" (doctoral dissertation, University of Marburg, 1947), p. 53 and table, "Ausländische Studierende der Medizin und Zahnmedizin in Deutschland, s.s. 1911–w.s. 1935–36." For Russian women studying medicine in Vienna, see Waltraud Heindl, "Ausländische Studentinnen an der Universität Wien vor dem ersten Weltkrieg," *Wegenetz europäischen Geistes II: Universitäten und Studenten*, ed. Richard G. Plaschka and Karlheinz Mack (Munich: R. Oldenbourg, 1987), pp. 317–343. See, too, Jaroslav Ščapov, "Russische Studenten an den westeuropäischen Hochschulen," *Wegenetz europäischen Geistes: Wissenschaftszentren und geistige Wechselbeziehungen zwischen Mittel- und Südosteuropa vom Ende des 18. Jahrhunderts bis zum Ersten Weltkrieg*, ed. R. G. Plaschka and K. Mack (Munich: R. Oldenbourg, 1983), p. 396.
4. Dudgeon, "Women and Higher Education in Russia," p. 258.
5. In 1906, a total of 895 women were enrolled in medical schools in the United States. Mary Roth Walsh, *"Doctors Wanted: No Women Need Apply"*:

*Sexual Barriers in the Medical Profession, 1835–1975* (New Haven: Yale University Press, 1977), table 8, p. 240.

6. Jeanette E. Tuve, *The First Russian Women Physicians* (Newtonville, Mass.: Oriental Research Partners, 1984), p. 123. The 43 percent figure is taken from Ruth Dudgeon, "The Forgotten Minority: Women Students in Imperial Russia, 1872–1917," *Russian History/Histoire Russe*, 1982, *9:* 10.

7. Dudgeon, "Women and Higher Education in Russia," pp. 389–390.

8. Kaethe Schirmacher, *The Modern Woman's Rights Movement: A Historical Survey*, 2nd ed. (New York: Macmillan, 1912), p. 216.

9. Tuve, *First Russian Women Physicians*, p. 122.

10. Ann H. Koblitz, *A Convergence of Lives: Sofia Kovalevskaia, Scientist, Writer, Revolutionary* (Boston: Birkhauser, 1983), p. ix.

11. Sergei Svatikov, "Russkaia studentka: 1860–1915," in *Put' studenchestva* (Moscow, 1916), p. 2. This is a collection of essays reprinted from the student fortnightly paper *Put' studenchestva* (Petrograd) of the previous year.

12. G. M. Grebenshchikov in an article of 1883 cited by Genia Adirim, *Das medizinische Frauenstudium in Russland* (Berlin: Freie Universität, 1984), pp. 29–30.

13. Quoted in Richard Stites, *The Women's Liberation Movement in Russia: Feminism, Nihilism, and Bolshevism, 1860–1930* (Princeton: Princeton University Press, 1978), p. 100.

14. Ann H. Koblitz, "Science, Women, and the Russian Intelligentsia: The Generation of the 1860s," *Isis*, 1988, *79:* 208.

15. Cynthia H. Whittaker, "The Women's Movement during the Reign of Alexander II: A Case Study in Russian Liberalism," *Journal of Modern History*, 1976, on demand supplement, *48:* 37.

16. Stites, *Women's Liberation Movement in Russia*, p. 51.

17. Whittaker, "Women's Movement during the Reign of Alexander II," p. 38.

18. L. F. Panteleev, *Vospominaniia* (Moscow, 1958), p. 214.

19. Svatikov, "Russkaia Studentka," p. 4.

20. Vasilii Teplov, "Piatidesiatiletie vysshago zhenskago obrazovaniia v Rossii," *Vestnik vospitaniia*, 1910, *9:* 119.

21. A. V. Pavluchkova, "Bor'ba progressivnoi meditsinskoi obshchestvennosti za vvedenie zhenskogo vrachebnogo obrazovaniia v Rossii (60-e-nachalo 70 kh godov xix veka," *Sovetskoe zdravookhranenia*, 1976, *4:* 60.

22. Teplov, "Piatidesiatiletie vysshago zhenskago obrazovania," p. 124.

23. Svatikov, "Russkaia Studentka," p. 5.

24. Dudgeon, "Women and Higher Education in Russia," p. 36.

25. Svatikov, "Russkaia Studentka," p. 5.

26. Stites, *Women's Liberation Movement in Russia*, p. 53.

27. This account of Kashevarova's life is based on the biography by Semen M. Dionesov, *V. A. Kashevarova-Rudneva—pervaia russkaia zhenshchina-doktor meditsiny* (Moscow, 1965), pp. 20–23.

28. Ibid., pp. 26–30.

29. Tuve, *First Russian Women Physicians*, p. 49.

30. Ibid.

31. Dionesov, *V. A. Kashevarova-Rudneva*, pp. 38–50.

32. Tuve, *First Russian Women Physicians,* pp. 50–51.

33. Dudgeon, "Women and Higher Education in Russia," p. 65.

34. Barbara A. Engel, "Women Medical Students in Russia, 1872–1882: Reformers or Rebels?" *Journal of Social History,* 1978, *12:* 398.

35. Dudgeon, "Women and Higher Education in Russia," pp. 65–66.

36. Adirim, *Das medizinische Frauenstudium,* p. 33.

37. S. M. Dionesov, "Russkie tsiurikhskie studentki-medichki v revoliutsionnom dvizhenii 70-kh godov xix stoletiia," *Sovetskoe zdravookhranenie,* 1973, *11:* 68.

38. Teplov, "Piatidesiatiletie vysshago zhenskago obrazovania," p. 126.

39. Stites, *Women's Liberation Movement in Russia,* p. 77.

40. Svatikov, "Russkaia studentka," p. 9.

41. The most thorough treatments of these developments are found in Dudgeon, "Women and Higher Education in Russia," pp. 103–106, and Christine Johanson, *Women's Struggle for Higher Education in Russia, 1855–1900* (Kingston and Montreal: McGill-Queen's University Press, 1987), pp. 77–81.

42. Svatikov, "Russkaia studentka," p. 13.

43. E. S. Nekrasova, "Zhenskie vrachebnye kursy v Peterburge," *Vestnik Evropy,* 1882, *6:* 817–818.

44. Ibid., p. 847; Svatikov, "Russkaia studentka," p. 13.

45. Tuve, *First Russian Women Physicians,* pp. 62–64.

46. Ibid., pp. 59–73.

47. These data were given by Dr. W. Kernig, chief of the women's hospital in St. Petersburg, to Arthur Kirchoff in 1897: *Die akademische Frau: Gutachten hervorragender Universitätsprofessoren, Frauenlehrer und Schriftsteller über die Befähigung der Frau zum wissenschaftlichen Studium und Berufe* (Berlin: Hugo Steinitz, 1897), table, p. 362.

48. Caroline Schultze, *Die Aerztin im XIX. Jahrhundert* (Leipzig: Peter Hobbing, 1889), p. 33.

49. F. Erismann, "Khodataistva Pravleniia ob otkrytii vysshikh zhenskikh kursov i o pravakh zhenshchin vrachei, obuchavshikhsia zagranitsei," *Zhurnal obshchestva russkikh vrachei v pamiat N. I. Pirogova* (Moscow), 1895, *1:* 15–21.

50. Nekrasova, "Zhenskie vrachebnye kursy," p. 640.

51. Adirim, *Das medizinische Frauenstudium in Russland,* p. 70.

52. Engel, "Women Medical Students in Russia," p. 406.

53. Tuve, *First Russian Women Physicians,* p. 66; Adirim, *Das medizinische Frauenstudium in Russland,* p. 99.

54. Tuve, p. 67.

55. Stites, *Women's Liberation Movement in Russia,* p. 87.

56. Engel, "Women Medical Students in Russia," p. 406.

57. A. I. Malozemova, "Zhenshchiny-mediki v politi-cheskikh protsessakh 1881 g. (k 100-letiiu protsessov)," *Sovetskoe Zdravookhranenie,* 1881, *7:* 54–59.

58. Dionesov, "Russkie tsiurikhskie studentki-medichki," pp. 68–71.

59. Engel, "Women Medical Students in Russia," p. 408.

60. Adirim, *Das medizinische Frauenstudium in Russland,* pp. 91–133; Dudgeon, "Women and Higher Education in Russia," pp. 192–223.

61. Adirim, *Das medizinische Frauenstudium in Russland,* pp. 94–96.

62. Daniela Neumann, *Studentinnen aus dem Russischen Reich in der Schweiz (1867–1914)* (Zurich: Hans Rohr, 1987), p. 201.

63. Jaroslav N. Ščapov found seven such books that appeared in the years 1898–1911: "Russische Studenten an den westeuropäischen Hochschulen," p. 396.

64. Alfred E. Senn, *The Russian Revolution in Switzerland, 1914–1917* (Madison: University of Wisconsin Press, 1971), p. 6.

65. Adirim, *Das medizinische Frauenstudium in Russland*, pp. 101–111.

66. Erismann, "Khodataistva Pravleniia ob otkrytii vysshikh zhenskikh kursov," pp. 15–21. For a biography of Erismann, see Hanspeter Wick, *Friedrich Huldreich Erismann (1842–1915): Russischer Hygieniker—Zürcher Stadtrat* (Zurich: Zürcher Medizingeschichtliche Abhandlungen, n.s. 82, 1970).

67. Dudgeon, "Women and Higher Education in Russia," p. 252.

68. Tuve, *First Russian Women Physicians*, pp. 111–112; Adirim, *Das medizinische Frauenstudium in Russland*, p. 117.

69. Adirim, *Das medizinische Frauenstudium in Russland*, pp. 115–122.

70. Dudgeon, "The Forgotten Minority," pp. 16–20.

71. Ibid., pp. 2–8; and Dudgeon, "Women and Higher Education in Russia," pp. 299–303.

72. Tuve, *First Russian Women Physicians*, pp. 114–117.

73. Dudgeon, "The Forgotten Minority," p. 13.

74. Friedrich Erismann, "Das medizinische Studium und die ärztliche Praxis der Frauen," *Die Frau*, 1893–94, *1*: 747–749; Raymond Hollmann, "Die Stellungnahme der Ärzte im Streit um das Medizinstudium der Frau bis zum Beginn des 20. Jahrhunderts" (doctoral dissertation, University of Münster, 1976), pp. 87–88.

75. Tuve, *First Russian Women Physicians*, p. 122.

76. Neumann, *Studentinnen aus dem Russischen Reich*, pp. 181–182.

77. Siegfried Rosenfeld, "Das Medizinstudium der Frauen in der Gegenwart," *Wiener Medizinische Blätter*, 1896, *19*: 7–8.

## 5. Imperial Germany

1. J. Schwalbe, *Über das medizinische Frauenstudium in Deutschland* (Leipzig: Georg Thieme, 1918), pp. 42–43.

2. Elisabeth Burger, "Die Entwicklung des medizinischen Frauenstudiums" (doctoral dissertation, University of Marburg, 1947), p. 53.

3. Elke Rupp, *Der Beginn des Frauenstudiums an der Universität Tübingen* (Tübingen: Universitätsarchiv, 1978), p. 26.

4. James C. Albisetti, "The Fight for Female Physicians in Imperial Germany," *Central European History*, 1982, *15*: 101.

5. Gordon A. Craig, *The Germans* (New York: New American Library, 1982), p. 147.

6. Agnes C. Vietor, ed., *A Woman's Quest: The Life of Marie E. Zakrzewska, M.D.* (New York: D. Appleton, 1924), p. 46.

7. Helene Lange, *Higher Education of Women in Europe* (New York: D. Appleton, 1890), p. 2.

8. Ibid., pp. 152–156.

9. Christine Eckelmann and Kristin Hoesch, "Ärztinnen—Emanzipation durch den Krieg?" *Medizin und Krieg: vom Dilemma der Heilberufe 1865 bis 1985,* ed. Johanna Bleker and Heinz-Peter Schmiedebach (Berlin: Fischer Taschenbuch Verlag, [1985]), pp. 155–156.

10. Kaethe Schirmacher, *The Modern Woman's Rights Movement* (New York: Macmillan, 1912), pp. 158–163.

11. Anna Schepeler-Lette and Jenny Hirsch, "Germany," in *The Woman Question in Europe,* ed. Theodore Stanton (New York: G. P. Putnam's Sons, 1884), p. 143.

12. Hugh W. Puckett, *Germany's Women Go Forward* (New York: Columbia University Press, 1930), p. 180.

13. Antke Luhn, "Geschichte des Frauenstudiums an der medizinischen Fakultät der Universität Göttingen" (doctoral disseration, University of Göttingen, 1971), p. 6. On the training of teachers, see Maria W. Blochmann, *Lass dich gelüsten nach der Männer Weisheit und Bildung* (Pfaffenweiler: Centaurus, 1990).

14. Siegfried Rosenfeld, "Das Medizinstudium der Frauen in der Gegenwart," *Wiener medizinische Blätter,* 1896, *19:* 9; see, too, Laetitia Boehm, "Von den Anfängen des akademischen Frauenstudiums in Deutschland: Zugleich ein Kapitel aus der Geschichte der Ludwig-Maximilians-Universität München," *Historisches Jahrbuch,* 1958, *77:* 298–327.

15. Konrad H. Jarausch, *Students, Society, and Politics in Imperial Germany: The Rise of Academic Illiberalism* (Princeton: Princeton University Press, 1982), p. 110.

16. M. Carey Thomas to Eva Channing, 24 September 1879, New England Hospital Collection, Box 21, folder 1107, Sophia Smith Collection, Smith College, Northampton, Massachusetts.

17. "The Contributors' Club," *Atlantic Monthly,* 1879, *44:* 789.

18. Sonja Brentjes and Karl-Heinz Schlote, "Zum Frauen-studium an der Universität Leipzig in der Zeit von 1870 bis 1910," in *Perspektiven interkultureller Wechselwirkung für den wissenschaftlichen Fortschritt,* Akademie der Wissenschaften der DDR Kolloquien, Heft 48 (Berlin: Nationalkomitee für Geschichte und Philosophie der Wissenschaften, 1985), pp. 24–25. See, too, Renate Drucker, "Zur Vorgeschichte des Frauenstudiums an der Universität Leipzig," in *Vom Mittelalter zur Neuzeit,* ed. Hellmut Kretzschmar (Berlin: Rütten & Loening, 1956), pp. 278–282.

19. Luhn, "Geschichte des Frauenstudiums," p. 20.

20. Walther Schönfeld, "Die Einstellung der Heidelberger medizinischen Fakultät in den achtziger Jahren zum Medizinstudium der Frauen," *Rupert-Carola,* 1961, *29:* 199.

21. Theodor von Bischoff, *Das Studium und die Ausübung der Medicin durch Frauen* (Munich: Literarisch-Artistische Anstalt, 1872), p. 41.

22. Franziska Tiburtius, *Erinnerungen einer Achtzigjährigen,* 3rd ed. (Berlin: C. A. Schwetschke, 1929), p. 132.

23. James C. Albisetti, *Schooling German Girls and Women: Secondary and Higher Education in the Nineteenth Century* (Princeton: Princeton University Press, 1988), pp. 123–125.

24. Tiburtius, *Erinnerungen,* p. 108.

25. Schweizerischer Verband der Akademikerinnen, *Das Frauenstudium an den Schweizer Hochschulen* (Zurich: Rascher, 1928), p. 61.

26. Franziska Tiburtius, "The Development of the Study of Medicine for Women in Germany, and Present Status," *Canadian Practitioner and Review,* 1909, *34:* 493.

27. Burger, "Die Entwicklung des medizinischen Frauenstudiums," p. 49.

28. Gustav Cohn, "Die deutsche Frauenbewegung," *Deutsche Rundschau,* 1896, *86:* 410.

29. Hanny Rohner, *Die ersten 30 Jahre des medizinischen Frauenstudiums an der Universität Zurich, 1867–1897* (Zürich: Juris Druck & Verlag, 1972), pp. 88–89; Tiburtius, *Erinnerungen,* p. 218.

30. Matrikel der Universität Zürich 1833–1933, Staatsarchiv, Zurich.

31. Rohner, *Die ersten 30 Jahre,* p. 42.

32. Burger, "Die Entwicklung des medizinischen Frauenstudiums," pp. 45–46; K. Sablik, "Zum Beginn des Frauenstudiums an der Wiener medizinischen Fakultät," *Wiener medizinische Wochenschrift,* 1968, *118:* 3.

33. See Marlene Jantsch, "Der Aufstieg der österreichischen Ärztin zur Gleichberechtigung," in *Frauenstudium und akademische Frauenarbeit in Österreich,* ed. martha Forkl and Elisabeth Koffmann (Vienna, 1968), and Karen J. Freeze, "Medical Education for Women in Austria: A Study in the Politics of the Czech Women's Movement in the 1890s," in *Women, State, and Party in Eastern Europe,* ed. Sharon L. Wolchik and Alfred G. Meyer (Durham: Duke University Press, 1985).

34. L. Henius, "Ueber die Zulassung der Frauen zum Studium der Medicin," *Deutsche medicinische Wochenschrift,* 1895, *21:* 615.

35. Luhn, "Geschichte des Frauenstudiums," p. 68.

36. Frances Elizabeth Hoggan, "Women in Medicine," in *The Woman Question in Europe,* ed. Theodore Stanton (New York: G. P. Putnam's Sons, 1884), pp. 85–86.

37. Victor Böhmert, *Das Studieren der Frauen mit besonderer Rücksicht auf das Studium der Medecin* (Leipzig: Otto Wigand, 1872), pp. 6–7.

38. W. von Zehender, *Ueber den Beruf der Frauen zum Studium und zur praktischen Ausbildung der Heilwissenschaft* (Rostock: Stiller'sche Hof- und Universitätsbuchhandlung, 1875), p. 22.

39. Marjorie H. Dobkin, ed., *The Making of a Feminist: Early Journals and Letters of M. Carey Thomas* (Kent, Ohio: Kent State University Press, 1979), p. 232.

40. P. J. Möbius, *Über den physiologischen Schwachsinn des Weibes,* 3rd ed. (Halle: Carl Marhold, 1901), pp. 4ff.

41. E. Albert, *Die Frauen und das Studium der Medicin* (Vienna: Alfred Hölder, 1895), p. 21.

42. Henius, "Ueber die Zulassung der Frauen," p. 613.

43. H. Fehling, *Die Bestimmung der Frau: Ihre Stellung zu Familie und Beruf* (Stuttgart: Ferdinand Enke, 1892), p. 15.

44. Raymond Hollmann, "Die Stellungnahme der Ärzte im Streit um das Medizinstudium der Frau bis zum Beginn des 20. Jahrhunderts" (doctoral

dissertation, University of Münster, 1976), p. 45.

45. Arthur Kirchoff, *Die akademische Frau: Gutachten hervorragenden Universitätsprofessoren, Frauenlehrer und Schriftsteller über die Befähigung der Frau zum wissenschaftlichen Studium und Berufe* (Berlin: Hugo Steinitz, 1897), p. 77.

46. Fehling, *Bestimmung der Frau,* p. 17.

47. Hollman, "Stellungnahme der Ärzte," p. 62.

48. See Kirchoff, *Die akademische Frau,* p. 47.

49. Ibid., pp. 71, 112.

50. Friedrich Erismann, "Das medizinische Studium und die ärztliche Praxis der Frauen," *Die Frau,* 1893–94, *1:* 747–749.

51. A. Jacobi, "Das medicinische Frauenstudium in Amerika," *Deutsche medicinische Wochenschrift,* 1896, *22:* 403.

52. Erika Ganss, "Die Entwicklung des Frauenmedizinstudium an deutschen Universitäten unter besonderer Berücksichtigung der Philipps-Universität in Marburg" (doctoral dissertation, University of Marburg, 1983), p. 43.

53. Kirchoff, *Die akademische Frau,* pp. 123–124.

54. Tiburtius, *Erinnerungen,* pp. 172–173.

55. James C. Albisetti, "Could Separate Be Equal? Helene Lange and Women's Education in Imperial Germany," *History of Education Quarterly,* 1982, *22:* 305.

56. Richard J. Evans, *The Feminist Movement in Germany, 1894–1933* (London: Sage Publications, 1976), p. 35.

57. Cohn, "Die Deutsche Frauenbewegung," p. 412.

58. Mathilde Weber, *Ärztinnen für Frauenkrankheiten: Eine ethische und eine sanitäre Notwendigkeit* (Tübingen, 1888).

59. Mathilde Weber, *Ein Besuch in Zürich bei den weiblichen Studierenden der Medizin* (Stuttgart: W. Kohlhammer, 1888), pp. 4–9.

60. Albisetti, "The Fight for Female Physicians," p. 107n.

61. Ibid., pp. 115–119. Albisetti's account of these developments is by far the most thorough and reliable.

62. J. Steudel, "Medical Women of the Occident," *Journal of the American Medical Women's Association,* 1962, *17:* 52. This article was translated from the *Zentralblatt für Gynäkologie,* 1959, *81:* 284–295.

63. Albisetti, *Schooling German Girls and Women,* pp. 223–224. The Americans included Abby Leach, Mary Calkins, Ida Keller, Jane Sherzer, Ellen Semple, Adele Luxenburg, Isabelle Bronk, Ellen Clune, Georgianna Morrill, and Alice Walton.

64. Luhn, "Geschichte des Frauenstudiums," pp. 27–29, 71–79.

65. Regine Zott, "Zu den Anfängen des Frauenstudiums an der Berliner Universität," in *Perspektiven interkultureller Wechselwirkung für den wissenschaftlichen Fortschritt,* Akademie der Wissenschaften der DDR Kolloquien, Heft 48 (Berlin: Nationalkomitee für Geschichte und Philosophie der Wissenschaften, 1985), pp. 31–33.

66. E. Th. Nauck, *Das Frauenstudium an der Universität Freiburg I. Br.* (Freiburg: Eberhard Albert Universitätsbuchhandlung, 1953), pp. 14–25.

67. A. Eulenberg, "Das Medizinstudium der Frauen an den deutschen Universitäten im Sommersemester 1901," *Deutsche medicinische Wochenschrift,* 1901, *27:* 472.
68. Isabel Maddison, *Handbook of Courses Open to Women in British, Continental and Canadian Universities* (New York: Macmillan, 1896), pp. 53–76.
69. Puckett, *Germany's Women Go Forward,* p. 188; Eulenburg, "Das Medizinstudium der Frauen," p. 472.
70. Elisabeth Platzer, "Frau Dr. med. Ilse Szagunn zum 80. Geburtstag," *Münchener medizinische Wochenschrift,* 1967, *109:* 1914.
71. *Deutsche illustrirte Zeitung,* 1895, p. 889. For good accounts of Linden's complicated career at Tübingen, see Elke Rupp, *Der Beginn des Frauenstudiums an der Universität Tübingen* (Tübingen: Universitätsarchiv, 1978), pp. 32–43, and Gabriele Junginger, ed., *Maria Gräfin von Linden: Erinnerungen der ersten Tübinger Studentin* (Tübingen: Attempto, 1991).
72. Ida H. Hyde, "Before Women Were Human Beings . . . Adventures of an American Fellow in German Universities of the '90s," *Journal of the American Association of University Women,* 1937–1939, *31–32:* 226–234.
73. Albisetti, "The Fight for Female Physicians," p. 112.
74. *Wiener medizinische Wochenschrift,* 1903, *16:* 765–769.
75. Cohn, "Die deutsche Frauenbewegung," p. 415.
76. Kirchhoff, *Die akademische Frau,* passim.
77. I am indebted to Professor James Albisetti for this quotation in a letter of 13 June 1990.
78. Franziska Tiburtius, "Frauenuniversitäten oder gemeinsames Studium?" *Die Frau,* 1898, *5:* 577–585.
79. Friedrich Erismann, *Gemeinsames Universitätsstudium für Männer und Frauen, oder besondere Frauen-Hochschulen?* Reprinted from *Die Frau,* 1899, *9–10.*
80. Ganss, "Entwicklung des Frauenstudiums," pp. 36–38.
81. Eulenberg, "Das Medizinstudium der Frauen," p. 472.
82. Ganss, "Entwicklung des Frauenstudiums," p. 38.
83. Abraham Flexner, *Medical Education in Europe: A Report to the Carnegie Foundation for the Advancement of Teaching* (New York: Carnegie Foundation for the Advancement of Teaching, Bulletin no. 6, 1912), p. 324.
84. Julius Pagel, *Grundriss eines Systems der medizinischen Kulturgeschichte* (Berlin, 1905), p. 43.
85. Cora B. Lattin, "The Woman Physician in Foreign Clinics," *Woman's Medical Journal,* 1910, *20:* 82.
86. Luhn, "Geschichte des Frauenstudiums," p. 60.
87. J. Schwalbe, *Über das medizinische Frauenstudium in Deutschland* (Leipzig: Georg Thieme, 1918), p. 16.
88. Burger, "Entwicklung des medizinischen Frauenstudiums," p. 53.
89. Schwalbe, *Über das medizinische Frauenstudium,* p. 42.
90. Konrad H. Jarausch, *Students, Society, and Politics in Imperial Germany: The Rise of Academic Illiberalism* (Princeton: Princeton University Press, 1982), p. 109.

91. James C. Albisetti, "Women and the Professions in Imperial Germany," in *German Women in the Eighteenth and Nineteenth Centuries: A Social and Literary History,* ed. Ruth-Ellen B. Joeres and Mary Jo Maynes (Bloomington: Indiana University Press, 1986), p. 104.

92. Ganss, "Entwicklung des Frauenstudiums," p. 56.

93. Aug. Fickert, "Das Medicinstudium der Frauen," *Wiener klinische Rundschau,* 1899, *13:* 241–243.

94. Jarausch, *Students, Society, and Politics in Imperial Germany,* pp. 64–65.

95. Luhn, "Geschichte des Frauenstudiums," pp. 41–42.

96. Brentjes and Schlote, "Zum Frauen-studium an der Universität Leipzig," p. 27.

97. Burger, "Entwicklung des medizinischen Frauenstudiums," table, "Ausländische Studierende der Medizin und Zahnmedizin in Deutschland, s.s. 1911–w.s. 1935/36."

98. Eckelmann and Hoesch, "Ärztinnen-Emanzipation durch den Krieg?" p. 158.

99. Ibid., p. 160.

100. Schwalbe, *Über das medizinische Frauenstudium,* p. 36.

## 6. The Fight for Coeducation in Britain

1. "Co-Education in Medical Colleges," *Woman's Medical Journal,* 1901, *11:* 13–14.

2. Elizabeth Smith, *"A Woman with a Purpose": The Diaries of Elizabeth Smith, 1872–1884,* ed. Veronica Strong-Boag (Toronto: University of Toronto Press, 1980), pp. xxiv–xxviii.

3. Mary Putnam Jacobi, "Woman in Medicine," in *Woman's Work in America,* ed. Annie Nathan Meyer (New York: Henry Holt, 1891), p. 199.

4. Martha L. Hildreth, "Delicacy and Propriety: The Acceptance of the Woman Physician in Victorian America," *Halcyon,* 1987, *9:* 152–153.

5. Emily F. Pope, Emma L. Call, and C. Augusta Pope, *The Practice of Medicine by Women in the United States* (Boston: Wright & Potter, 1881), pp. 1, 10.

6. Paige Kelly, "Upstarts: Opposition Greeted First Women Medical Students," *Advance* (University of Michigan School of Medicine), summer 1982, p. 4.

7. Smith, *Diaries of Elizabeth Smith,* p. 275.

8. Emily L. B. Forster, *How to Become a Woman Doctor* (London: Charles Griffin & Co., 1918), p. 52.

9. Jacobi, "Women in Medicine," p. 176.

10. Mary Roth Walsh, *"Doctors Wanted: No Women Need Apply": Sexual Barriers in the Medical Profession, 1835–1975* (New Haven: Yale University Press, 1977), p. 70.

11. Sophia Jex-Blake, *Medical Women: A Thesis and a History* (Edinburgh: Oliphant, Anderson, & Ferrier, 1886), p. 54.

12. H. E. MacDermot, *Maude Abbott: A Memoir* (Toronto: Macmillan, 1941), p. 41.

13. Mary Putnam Jacobi, "Women in Medicine," in *What America Owes to Women*, ed. Lydia Hoyt Farmer (Buffalo: National Exposition Souvenir, 1893), p. 382.
14. Vincent Y. Bowditch, *Life and Correspondence of Henry Ingersoll Bowditch*, 2 vols. (Boston and New York: Houghton Mifflin, 1902), 2: 253.
15. Meryl S. Justin, "The Entry of Women into Medicine in America: Education and Obstacles, 1847–1910," *Synthesis*, 1978, 4: 38.
16. *Journal of the American Medical Association*, 1883, 1: 183.
17. Regina M. Morantz-Sanchez, *Sympathy and Science: Women Physicians in American Medicine* (New York: Oxford University Press, 1985), p. 71.
18. Walsh, *"Doctors Wanted,"* table 8, p. 240.
19. Mary Ann C. Elston to author, 12 August 1988. See, too, her "Women Doctors in the British Health Service: A Sociological Study of Their Careers and Opportunities" (doctoral dissertation, University of London, 1986).
20. Helene Lange, *Higher Education of Women in Europe* (New York: D. Appleton, 1890), p. 42.
21. For the development of higher education for women in Great Britain, see Rhama D. Pope, "The Development of Formal Higher Education for Women in England, 1862–1914" (doctoral dissertation, University of Pennsylvania, 1972); S. Hamilton, "Women and the Scottish Universities circa 1869–1939: A Social History" (doctoral dissertation, University of Edinburgh, 1987), pp. 12–139; and Ray Strachey, *"The Cause": A Short History of the Women's Movement in Great Britain* (Port Washington, N.Y.: Kennikat Press, 1969), esp. pp. 124–186.
22. L. Martindale, *A Woman Surgeon* (London: Victor Gollancz, 1951), p. 32.
23. Elizabeth Sahli, "Elizabeth Blackwell, M.D. (1821–1910): A Biography" (doctoral dissertation, University of Pennsylvania, 1974), p. 217.
24. Jo Manton, *Elizabeth Garrett Anderson* (New York: E. P. Dutton, 1965), p. 128.
25. Strachey, *"The Cause,"* p. 175.
26. Margaret Todd, *The Life of Sophia Jex-Blake* (London: Macmillan, 1918), pp. 189n, 199–209. Dr. Lucy Sewall wrote after Jex-Blake's return to England because of her father's death: "If you don't come back to America, you won't give up the work. You will open the profession to women in England" (p. 209).
27. Jex-Blake, *Medical Women*, p. 69.
28. Hamilton, "Women and the Scottish Universities," p. 31. The following account of the women's struggle at Edinburgh is based principally on this work, Jex-Blake's *Medical Women*, E. Moberly Bell's *Storming the Citadel* (London: Constable, 1953), and Edythe Lutzker's *Women Gain a Place in Medicine* (New York: McGraw-Hill, 1969).
29. Isabel Thorne, *Sketch of the Foundation and Development of the London School of Medicine for Women* (London: G. Sharron, 1905), p. 5.
30. Jex-Blake, *Medical Women*, p. 79.
31. A. H. Bennett, *English Medical Women* (London: Sir Isaac Pitman & Sons, 1915), p. 19.

32. Jex-Blake, *Medical Women*, p. 92.
33. Thorne, *Sketch of . . . the London School of Medicine*, p. 9.
34. This account is from Strachey, "*The Cause*," p. 179.
35. Lutzker, *Women Gain a Place*, pp. 85–87.
36. Jex-Blake, *Medical Women*, p. 161.
37. Frances Elizabeth Hoggan, "Women in Medicine," in *The Woman Question in Europe*, ed. Theodore Stanton (New York and London: G. P. Putnam's Sons, 1884), pp. 71–72. Frances Morgan had married Dr. George Hoggan in 1874, four years after her return from Zurich.
38. Hamilton, "Women and the Scottish Universities," pp. 434–435.
39. Wilhelm von Zehender, *Ueber den Beruf der Frauen zum Studium und zur praktischen Ausbildung der Heilwissenschaft* (Rostock: Stiller'sche Hof- und Universitätsbuchhandlung, 1875), p. 30.
40. This account borrows from Joan N. Burstyn, "Education and Sex: The Medical Case against Higher Education for Women in England, 1870–1900," *Proceedings of the American Philosophical Society*, 1973, *117*: 79–89.
41. Edward H. Clarke, *Sex in Education; or, A Fair Chance for the Girls* (Boston: James R. Osgood, 1874), p. 39.
42. Ibid., pp. 23–24.
43. Sophia Jex-Blake, *A Visit to Some American Schools and Colleges* (London: Macmillan, 1867), p. 243.
44. See Hildreth, "Delicacy and Propriety," pp. 153–155.
45. Dorothy G. McGuigan, *A Dangerous Experiment: 100 Years of Women at the University of Michigan* (Ann Arbor: Center for Continuing Education of Women, 1970), p. 56.
46. William Goodell, *The Dangers and Duties of the Hour* (Baltimore: J. W. Borst, 1881), p. 3.
47. Elizabeth Fee, "Science and the 'Woman Question,' 1860–1920: A Study of English Scientific Periodicals" (doctoral dissertation, Princeton University, 1978), p. 205.
48. Manton, *Elizabeth Garrett Anderson*, pp. 232–233, 240.
49. Sahli, "Elizabeth Blackwell," p. 217.
50. Christopher St. John, *Christine Murrell, M.D.: Her Life and Her Work* (London: Williams & Norgate, 1935), pp. 25–26.
51. Ibid., p. 25.
52. Jex-Blake, *Medical Women*, p. 179.
53. Thorne, *Sketch of . . . the London School of Medicine*, p. 19; E. Moberly Bell, *Storming the Citadel* (London: Constable, 1953), p. 95.
54. Jex-Blake, *Medical Women*, pp. 168–220.
55. Caroline Schultze, *Die Aerztin im XIX Jahrhundert* (Leipzig: Peter Hobbing, 1889), pp. 44–45.
56. Manton, *Elizabeth Garrett Anderson*, pp. 109–110.
57. See London School of Medicine for Women, *Prospectus, 1886–87*.
58. London School of Medicine for Women, *Report, 1890*, pp. 8–28.
59. Martindale, *A Woman Surgeon*, pp. 32–33.
60. Wendy Alexander, *First Ladies of Medicine: The Origins, Education and Des-*

*tination of Early Women Medical Graduates of Glasgow University* (Glasgow: Wellcome Unit for the History of Medicine, 1988), pp. 4, 5–11. See, too, Hamilton, "Women and the Scottish Universities," pp. 128–129.

61. Alexander, *First Ladies*, pp. 12–20.
62. "The Scottish Universities Commission," *Lancet*, 1892, *1:* 661.
63. Hamilton, "Women and the Scottish Universities," p. 140.
64. Nan Shepherd, "Women in the University—Fifty Years: 1892–1942," *Aberdeen University Review*, 1941–42, *29:* 175–176.
65. Hamilton, "Women and the Scottish Universities," p. 149; R. D. Anderson, *Education and Opportunity in Victorian Scotland* (Oxford: Clarendon Press, 1983), p. 355.
66. Mary Ann Elston, "Women's Access to Medical Education in Great Britain, 1877–1900: An Overview," *Bulletin of the Society for the Social History of Medicine*, 1987, *41:* 53.
67. Hamilton, "Women and the Scottish Universities," p. 162.
68. A. Logan Turner, *History of the University of Edinburgh, 1883–1933* (Edinburgh: Oliver and Boyd, 1933), pp. 161–162.
69. Anderson, *Education and Opportunity in Victorian Scotland,* p. 353.
70. Abraham Flexner, *Medical Education in Europe* (New York: Carnegie Foundation for the Advancement of Teaching, Bulletin no. 6, 1912), p. 326n.
71. Hamilton, "Women and the Scottish Universities," p. 163.
72. Julie S. Gilbert, "Women at the English Civic Universities, 1880–1920" (doctoral dissertation, University of North Carolina, 1988), pp. 204–207.
73. Mabel Tylecote, *The Education of Women at Manchester University, 1883 to 1933* (Manchester: University of Manchester Press, 1941), p. 50.
74. Elston, "Women's Access to Medical Education," p. 51.
75. See the figures in Flexner, *Medical Education in Europe,* p. 325; the tables on Scottish enrollment in Anderson, *Education and Opportunity in Victorian Scotland,* pp. 352–356; and Tylecote, *Education of Women at Manchester University,* p. 55. But Mary Ann Elston, in a letter to the author, has emphasized how uncertain the pre-1914 data are.
76. See, e.g., Tylecote, *Education of Women at Manchester University,* pp. 135–138.

## 7. *America: Triumph and Paradox*

1. Regina M. Morantz-Sanchez, "Women Physicians, Coeducation, and the Struggle for Professional Standards in Nineteenth-Century Medical Education" (paper presented at Berkshire Conference on the History of Women, August 1978), pp. 3–7.
2. Sophia Jex-Blake, *A Visit to Some American Schools and Colleges* (London: Macmillan, 1867), p. 226.
3. Thomas Woody, *A History of Women's Education in the United States,* 2 vols. (New York: Science Press, 1929), *2:* 253.
4. Barbara M. Solomon, *In the Company of Educated Women: A History of Women and Higher Education in America* (New Haven: Yale University Press, 1985),

table 1, p. 44. See, too, Lynn D. Gordon, *Gender and Higher Education in the Progressive Era* (New Haven: Yale University Press, 1990), pp. 13–51.

5. Kaethe Schirmacher, *The Modern Woman's Rights Movement: A Historical Survey* (New York: Macmillan, 1912), pp. 96–97.

6. Elizabeth Smith, *"A Woman with a Purpose": The Diaries of Elizabeth Smith, 1872–1884,* ed. Veronica Strong-Boag (Toronto: University of Toronto Press, 1980), p. xxii.

7. MS of talk given 30 March 1883, New England Hospital Papers, Box 27, folder 1173, Sophia Smith Collection, Smith College, Northampton, Massachusetts.

8. John C. Gerber, *A Pictorial History of the University of Iowa* (Iowa City: University of Iowa Press, 1988), pp. 28, 43.

9. This paragraph relies heavily on Dorothy G. McGuigan, *A Dangerous Experiment: 100 Years of Women at the University of Michigan* (Ann Arbor: Center for Continuing Education for Women, 1970), pp. 20–37.

10. Ibid., p. 63.

11. Wilfred B. Shaw, ed., *The University of Michigan: An Encyclopedic Survey,* 4 vols. (Ann Arbor: University of Michigan Press, 1951), 2: 792.

12. Woody, *History of Women's Education,* 2: 246.

13. Paige Kelly, "Upstarts: Opposition Greeted First Women Medical Students," *Advance* (University of Michigan School of Medicine), summer 1982, p. 1.

14. Shaw, *University of Michigan,* 2: 792.

15. Agnes C. Vietor, ed., *A Woman's Quest: The Life of Marie E. Zakrzewska, M.D.* (New York: D. Appleton, 1924), p. 384.

16. Regina M. Morantz-Sanchez, *Sympathy and Science: Women Physicians in American Medicine* (New York: Oxford University Press, 1985), table 9-2, p. 245.

17. William Barlow and David O. Powell, "Homeopathy and Sexual Equality: The Controversy over Coeducation at Cincinnati's Pulte Medical College, 1873–1879," in *Women and Health in America,* ed. Judith W. Leavitt (Madison: University of Wisconsin Press, 1984), p. 422.

18. Harold J. Abrahams, *Extinct Medical Schools of Nineteenth-Century Philadelphia* (Philadelphia: University of Pennsylvania Press, 1966), pp. 288–331.

19. *Announcement of the Penn Medical College of Philadelphia, Female Session* (Philadelphia: G. S. Harris, 1853), p. 7.

20. William Barlow and David O. Powell, "A Case for Medical Coeducation in the 1870s," *Journal of the American Medical Women's Association,* 1980, *35:* 286–288.

21. Harold J. Abrahams, *The Extinct Medical Schools of Baltimore, Maryland* (Baltimore: Maryland Historical Society, 1969), p. 265.

22. Thomas F. Harrington, *The Harvard Medical School: A History, Narrative and Documentary,* 3 vols. (New York: Lewis Publishing Company, 1905), *3:* 1217.

23. "Majority Report," Harvard Medical School records, Countway Library, Harvard Medical School.

24. Agassiz to Mary Putnam Jacobi, 16 May 1878, Mary Putnam Jacobi Papers, Schlesinger Library, Radcliffe College.
25. Francis Minot to Edward Jarvis, 17 July 1878, Francis Minot Papers, Countway Library.
26. Agassiz to Mary Putnam Jacobi, 16 June 1879, Mary Putnam Jacobi Papers, Schlesinger Library.
27. Untitled, undated clipping, J. R. Chadwick Scrapbook, Women in Medicine Collection, Countway Library.
28. Harrington, *Harvard Medical School, 3:* 1243.
29. Selma H. Calmes, "Rose Talbot Bullard, MD: LACMA's Only Woman President," *Los Angeles County Medical Association Physician,* 17 October 1983, p. 27.
30. Unsigned letter to J. R. Chadwick, 12 June 1879, J. R. Chadwick Scrapbook, Countway Library, Harvard Medical School.
31. Robert H. Shikes and Henry N. Claman, *The University of Colorado School of Medicine: A Centennial History, 1883–1983* (Denver: Board of Regents of the University of Colorado, 1983), p. 85.
32. Carlotta Hacker, *The Indomitable Lady Doctors* (Toronto: Clarke, Irwin, 1974), pp. 56–65.
33. *Sixth Annual Calendar of the Women's Medical College, Kingston* (Kingston: British Whig Office, 1888), p. 2.
34. Hacker, *Indomitable Lady Doctors,* pp. 242–243.
35. *Seventh Annual Announcement of the Woman's Medical College Toronto, 1889–90* (Toronto: Brough & Caswell, 1889).
36. Hacker, *Indomitable Lady Doctors,* pp. 242–246.
37. See the list in Esther P. Lovejoy, *Women Doctors of the World* (New York: Macmillan, 1957), p. 120.
38. Printed list of graduates, New York Medical College and Hospital for Women, source unknown, Archives and Special Collections on Women in Medicine, Medical College of Pennsylvania, Philadelphia (hereafter cited as Archives and Special Collections).
39. *Annual Announcement of the Woman's Medical College and Woman's Hospital of St. Louis* (St. Louis, 1895).
40. *First Annual Announcement of the Woman's Medical College, Kansas City, Mo.* (Kansas City: Hudson-Kimberly, 1895).
41. James T. Whittaker to Clara Marshall, 19 October 1893, bound with *Announcement of the Woman's Medical College of Cincinnati, 1894–5* (Cincinnati, 1894), Archives and Special Collections.
42. Mary Putnam Jacobi, "Woman in Medicine," in *Woman's Work in America,* ed. Annie Nathan Meyer (New York: Henry Holt, 1891), p. 170n.
43. *Announcement of Presbyterian Hospital and Woman's Medical College, Cincinnati, 1894–95* (Cincinnati, 1894).
44. Printed list of graduates of Laura Memorial Woman's Medical College, Cincinnati, source unknown, Archives and Special Collections.
45. Woman's Medical College of Georgia, *First Annual Announcement* (Atlanta:

American Book and Job Print, 1889), pp. 6–7; "Society: A Journal Devoted to Society, Art, Literature, Fashion, Atlanta, Georgia, March 7, 1891," MS in Women's Medical Education file, American Medical Women's Association, Archives and Special Collections, p. 1.

46. Compiled from Alumnae Files, Woman's Medical College of Pennsylvania, Archives and Special Collections.

47. E. Clark to WMCP, undated, Archives and Special Collections.

48. Clara Marshall to Editor of *Illustrated London News*, 27 December 1907, Clara Marshall Papers, Archives and Special Collections, file C-4.

49. Iver C. Shattuck to Alice Stone Blackwell, 28 October 1889, Archives and Special Collections, file C-4.

50. Autobiography, chapter III, pp. 1–7, Anna Williams Papers, Carton 1, Schlesinger Library, Radcliffe College.

51. Helga M. Rudd, "The Women's [*sic*] Medical College of Chicago," *Medical Woman's Journal*, 1946, *53:* 46; Thomas N. Bonner, "Mary Harris Thompson," in *Notable American Women, 1607–1950*, ed. Edward T. James and Janet W. James, 3 vols. (Cambridge, Mass.: Belknap Press of Harvard University Press, 1971), *3:* 455–456.

52. Abrahams, *Extinct Medical Schools of Baltimore*, pp. 71–72, 109.

53. Steven J. Peitzman, "The Quiet Life of a Philadelphia Medical Woman: Mary Willits (1855–1902)," *Journal of the American Medical Women's Association*, 1979, *34:* 445–446.

54. Emily F. Pope, Emma L. Call, and C. Augusta Pope, *The Practice of Medicine by Women in the United States* (Boston: Wright & Potter, 1881), pp. 2–5.

55. Ruth J. Abram, ed., *"Send Us a Lady Physician": Women Doctors in America, 1835–1920* (New York: W. W. Norton, 1985), p. 132.

56. Virginia Drachman, "The Limits of Progress: The Professional Lives of Women Doctors, 1881–1926," *Bulletin of the History of Medicine*, 1986, *60:* 66.

57. Darlene Clark Hine, "Co-Laborers in the Work of the Lord: Nineteenth-Century Black Women Physicians," in Abram, *"Send Us a Lady Physician,"* p. 108.

58. Bettina Aptheker, *Woman's Legacy: Essays on Race, Sex, and Class in American History* (Amherst: University of Massachusetts Press, 1982), p. 100.

59. Hine, "Co-Laborers in the Work of the Lord," pp. 110–111.

60. Bureau of Census, *Fourteenth Census of the United States in the Year 1920, 4* (Washington: Government Printing Office, 1923): 737.

61. Frederick C. Waite, "Medical Education of Women in Cleveland (1850–1930)," *Western Reserve University Bulletin*, 1930, *16:* 16; Mary R. Walsh, *"Doctors Wanted: No Women Need Apply": Sexual Barriers in the Medical Profession, 1835–1975* (New Haven: Yale University Press, 1977), table 8, p. 240.

62. Clara J. Alexander, "A Forecast in Medical Education," *Transactions of the Alumnae Association of the Woman's Medical College of Pennsylvania*, 1905, *30:* 65.

63. "Women and Medicine," *Nation*, 1891, *52:* 131.
64. Woman's Medical College of the New York Infirmary for Women and Children, *Final Catalogue* [New York, 1899], p. 12.
65. "General Circular," text in Alan M. Chesney, *The Johns Hopkins Hospital and the Johns Hopkins University School of Medicine*, 3 vols. (Baltimore: Johns Hopkins Press, 1943–1963), *1:* 292.
66. Sarah H. Stevenson, "The Training and Qualifications of Women Doctors," in *Women in Professions*, International Congress of Women (London: T. Fisher Unwin, 1900), p. 51.
67. This information is derived from a variety of sources, including: Alumnae Association of the Woman's Medical College of Pennsylvania, *Transactions of the Twenty-Fifth Annual Meeting* (Philadelphia: Alumnae Association of WMCP, 1900); and "Co-Education in Medical Colleges," *Woman's Medical Journal*, 1901, *11:* 13.
68. Woman's Medical College of the New York Infirmary, *Final Catalogue*, pp. 7, 9.
69. Morantz-Sanchez, *Sympathy and Science*, p. 247.
70. Minutes of Faculty, Northwestern University Woman's Medical School, 6 June 1900, Northwestern University Woman's Medical School Records, Archives and Special Collections.
71. Bertha Van Hoosen, *Petticoat Surgeon* (Chicago: Pellegrini & Cudahy, 1947), pp. 137–138.
72. Abraham Flexner, *Medical Education in the United States and Canada* (New York: Carnegie Foundation for the Advancement of Teaching, Bulletin no. 4, 1910), pp. 179, 237, 271, 296.
73. John R. Abercrombie to Clara Marshall, 30 April 1910, Archives and Special Collections.
74. Abraham, *Extinct Medical Schools of Baltimore*, p. 73.
75. Clara Marshall to A. Flexner, 2 June 1909, Archives C-4, Clara Marshall Papers, folder 9, Archives and Special Collections.
76. N. P. Colwell to Annie W. Bosworth, 14 February 1913, Archives and Special Collections.
77. "Woman's Medical College of Pennsylvania, Inspected Dec. 9, 1913," MS, Clara Marshall Papers, folder 9, Archives and Special Collections.
78. Morantz-Sanchez, *Sympathy and Science*, pp. 255–259.
79. Stevenson, "Training and Qualifications of Women Doctors," p. 51.
80. Jacobi, "Woman in Medicine," p. 197.
81. Lydia Rabinowitsch, "Die amerikanische Frau und ihre Leistungen," *Die Frauenbewegung*, 1897, *3:* 4. For her career at the Woman's Medical College of Pennsylvania, see MS by Barbara Dewey, University of Michigan [1949], copy in Archives and Special Collections.
82. Gloria Moldow, *Women Doctors in Gilded-Age Washington* (Urbana: University of Illinois Press, 1987), p. 2.
83. Gordon, *Gender and Higher Education*, pp. 43–44. See, too, Patricia S. Butcher, *Education for Equality: Women's Rights Periodicals and Women's*

*Higher Education, 1849–1920* (Westport, Conn.: Greenwood Press, 1989), pp. 45–48.

84. Stow Persons, "The Decline of Homeopathy—The University of Iowa, 1876–1919," *Bulletin of the History of Medicine,* 1991, *65:* 87.
85. Shaw, *University of Michigan, 2:* 792.
86. Walsh, *"Doctors Wanted,"* table 6, p. 193.
87. Woody, *History of Women's Education, 2:* 322.
88. Jacobi, "Woman in Medicine," p. 197.
89. Sophia Jex-Blake, *Medical Women: A Thesis and a History* (Edinburgh: Oliphant, Anderson, & Ferrier, 1886), pp. 246–247.
90. Caroline Schultze, *Die Aerztin im XIX. Jahrhundert* (Leipzig: Peter Hobbing, 1889), p. 54. This work, written as a thesis at the University of Paris, was published in both French and German.
91. Compiled from reports in Alumnae Association of the Woman's Medical College of Pennsylvania, *Transactions of the Twenty-Fifth Annual Meeting* (Philadelphia: Alumnae Association, 1900).
92. I am indebted to Professor Ellen More for calling my attention to the *Census of Women Physicians* published by the American Women's Hospitals in 1918. By subtracting those who graduated after 1900 in the Census, and adding the estimated number who died in the period 1900–1918, I arrived at a figure of 3,396 women with medical degrees in 1900.
93. A list of the contract surgeons may be found in the American Medical Women's Association papers, Archives and Special Collections.
94. Ellen More, " 'A Certain Restless Ambition': Women Physicians and World War I," *American Quarterly,* 1989, *41:* 637.
95. *Philadelphia Evening Ledger,* 2 June 1915.
96. *Philadelphia Evening Bulletin,* 1915, undated clipping, Ricka Finkler file, Women Physicians box, Archives and Special Collections; Walsh, *"Doctors Wanted,"* p. 221.
97. "The Exclusion of Women Students from London Medical Schools," *JAMA,* 1929, *92:* 735.
98. *London (Royal Free Hospital) School of Medicine for Women,* London [1915], p. 3.
99. See the list in Emily L. B. Forster, *How to Become a Woman Doctor* (London: Charles Griffin, 1918), pp. 9–47.
100. Christopher St. John, *Christine Murrell, M.D.: Her Life and Her Work* (London: Williams & Norgate, 1935), p. 73.
101. Jacobi, "Woman in Medicine," pp. 198–199.

*Epilogue: Since 1914*

1. Erika Ganss, "Die Entwicklung des Frauenmedizinstudiums an deutschen Universitäten unter besonderer Berücksichtigung der Phillips-Universität in Marburg" (doctoral dissertation, University of Marburg, 1983), p. 66; Mabel Tylecote, *The Education of Women at Manchester University, 1833 to 1933*

(Manchester: University of Manchester Press, 1941), p. 100; Jeannette E. Tuve, *The First Russian Women Physicians* (Newtonville, Mass.: Oriental Research Partners, 1984), p. 117.

2. "The Deplorable London Situation," *Medical Woman's Journal*, 1928, *35:* 291.
3. Nan Shepherd, "Women in the University Fifty Years: 1892–1942," *Aberdeen University Review*, 1941–42, *29:* 179.
4. Untitled newspaper clipping, London, 22 March 1922, Archives and Special Collections, MCP.
5. Martha Tracy to Winifred Cullis, London School of Medicine for Women, 13 January 1921 (copy), Martha Tracy Papers, Archives and Special Collections, MCP.
6. Christine Eckelmann and Kristin Hoesch, "Ärztinnen—Emanzipation durch den Krieg?" *Medizin und Krieg: vom Dilemma der Heilberufe, 1865 bis 1915,* ed. Johanna Bleker and Heinz-Peter Schmiedebach (Fischer Taschenbuch Verlag, [1985]), p. 167.
7. Antke Luhn, "Geschichte des Frauenstudiums an der medizinischen Fakultät der Universität Göttingen" (doctoral dissertation, University of Göttingen, 1971), p. 99.
8. Kenneth Ludmerer, *Learning to Heal: The Development of American Medical Education* (New York: Basic Books, 1985), table 13.2, p. 248.
9. *The Pennsylvanian*, 14 February 1920.
10. Richard Stites, *The Women's Liberation Movement in Russia: Feminism, Nihilism, and Bolshevism, 1860–1930* (Princeton: Princeton University Press, 1978), p. 322.
11. Tuve, *First Russian Women Physicians*, p. 125. See, too, Michael Ryan, *Doctors and the State in the Soviet Union* (New York: St. Martin's Press, 1990).
12. *Annuaire statistique de la France, 1930,* p. 39.
13. Constance Joël, *Les filles d'Esculape: Les femmes à la conquête du pouvoir médical* (Paris: Robert Laffont, 1988), pp. 231–234.
14. The account in this paragraph and the following is based on the report of the London correspondent of the *Journal of the American Medical Association,* 1929. *92:* 735–736.
15. "Women in Medicine," *Journal of the American Medical Women's Association,* 1946, *1:* 93–94.
16. Kate C. Hurd-Mead, *Medical Women of America* (New York: Froben Press, 1933), p. 50.
17. Ibid., pp. 50–51.
18. Untitled newspaper clipping, Bertha Van Hoosen Papers, Bentley Library, University of Michigan.
19. See, e.g., Regina M. Morantz-Sanchez, *Sympathy and Science: Women Physicians in American Medicine* (New York: Oxford University Press, 1985), pp. 315–321.
20. Mary R. Walsh, *"Doctors Wanted: No Women Need Apply": Sexual Barriers in the Medical Profession, 1835–1975* (New Haven: Yale University Press, 1977), pp. 244–249.

21. Stephen Cole, "Sex Discrimination and Admission to Medical School, 1929–1984," *American Journal of Sociology,* 1986, *92:* 549–555.
22. William Pepper to Hans Zimmer, 18 May 1926, Countway Library, Harvard Medical School.
23. Ellen More, "The Blackwell Medical Society and the Professionalization of Women Physicians," *Bulletin of the History of Medicine,* 1987, *61:* 603.
24. Luhn, "Geschichte des Frauenstudiums," p. 99; Elisabeth Burger, "Entwicklung des medizinischen Frauenstudiums" (doctoral dissertation, University of Marburg, 1947), table, p. 69.
25. A. H. T. Robb-Smith, "The Fate of Oxford Medical Women," *Lancet,* 1 December 1962, p. 1160.
26. Fritz K. Ringer, *Education and Society in Modern Europe* (Bloomington: Indiana University Press, 1979), p. 67.
27. Burger, "Die Entwicklung des medizinischen Frauenstudiums," p. 68. See, too, the excellent discussion of medical women under the Nazis in Michael Kater, *Doctors under Hitler* (Chapel Hill: University of North Carolina Press, 1989), pp. 89–110.
28. Alice Hamilton, "Woman's Place in Germany," *Survey Graphic,* January 1934, p. 26.
29. Walsh, *"Doctors Wanted,"* p. 230.
30. *Philadelphia Inquirer,* 23 May 1941.
31. *New York Times,* 26 September 1945.
32. Ibid., 21 June 1942.
33. John Z. Bowers, "Women in Medicine: An International Study," *New England Journal of Medicine,* 1966, *275:* 362; Marjorie Galenson, *Women and Work: An International Comparison* (Ithaca, N.Y.: School of Industrial and Labor Relations, Cornell University, 1973), p. 24.
34. Information supplied by Medical Women's Federation, London, 28 June 1990.
35. Bowers, "Women in Medicine," p. 362.
36. Beverly C. Morgan, "Admission of Women into Medical Schools in the United States: Current Status," *Woman Physician,* 1971, *26:* 305.
37. Walsh, *"Doctors Wanted,"* p. 268.
38. "Enrollment in Canadian Faculties of Medicine by Sex, 1957/58–1989/90," information sent by Association of Canadian Medical Colleges, 24 May 1990.
39. Hilary Bourdillon, *Women as Healers: A History of Women and Medicine* (Cambridge: Cambridge University Press, 1988), p. 43.
40. Joël, *Les filles d'Esculape,* pp. 188–204, 227. See, too, J.-J. Bernier, "Croissance du corps médical," *Nouvelle presse médicale,* 1976, *5:* 517–519.
41. Information supplied by Mariella Böhme and the Bayerisches Landesamt für Statistik, 2 May 1991.
42. See, e.g., Joël, *Les filles d'Esculape,* pp. 204–219; Ruth J. Abram, ed., *"Send Us a Lady Physician": Women Doctors in America, 1835–1920* (New York: W. W. Norton, 1985), pp. 247–248; and A. P. Williams, K. Domnick-Pierre, E. Vayda, and M. Burke, "Women in Medicine: Practice Patterns and Attitudes," *Canadian Medical Association Journal,* 1990, *143:* 194–201.

# Bibliography

*Manuscripts and Other Unpublished Material*

*Ann Arbor.* Bentley Historical Library, University of Michigan
Mary T. Greene Papers
Eliza M. Mosher Papers
University of Michigan Medical School Faculty Minutes, 1850–1875
University of Michigan Regents Proceedings, 1864–1870
Bertha Van Hoosen Papers

*Bern.* Staatsarchiv Bern
Mappe der medizinischen Fakultät, Studierende, Frauenstudium, usw.

*Boston.* Boston University Library
Female Medical Education Society Record Book

*Boston.* Francis Countway Library
James R. Chadwick Scrapbook
Samuel Gregory Scrapbook
Harvard Medical School Papers
Francis Minot Papers
New England Female Medical College Scrapbook
Women in Medicine Collection

*Cambridge, Massachusetts.* Schlesinger Library, Radcliffe College
Mary Putnam Jacobi Papers
Margaret Noyes Kleinert Papers
Helen Morton Papers
New England Hospital for Women and Children Papers
Anna Wessel Williams Papers

*Northampton, Massachusetts.* Sophia Smith Collection, Smith College
Susan Dimock Letters
Dorothy Reed Mendenhall Papers
New England Hospital for Women and Children Papers

Schools and Societies Papers
Women Physicians Papers

*Paris.* Archives Nationales
Mary Putnam Dossier

*Philadelphia.* Archives and Special Collections on Women in Medicine, Medical College of Pennsylvania
Alumnae Files
American Medical Women's Association Papers
Rachel Bodley Papers
Sarah A. Hibbard Diary
Hannah Longshore Papers
Thomas E. Longshore Papers
Clara Marshall Papers
Northwestern University Woman's Medical School Records
Martha Tracy Papers
Woman's Hospital Medical College of Chicago Faculty Minutes
Woman's Medical College of Pennsylvania Records
Women Physicians Collection

*Zurich.* Medizinhistorisches Institut
August Forel Papers

*Zurich.* Staatsarchiv
Frauenstudium 1864–1879, Box U94 16
Matrikel der Universität Zürich

*Zurich.* University of Zurich Archives
Protokoll der medizinischen Fakultät Zürich, 1864–1890, 1890–1912
Senats-Protokoll, 1833–1880, 1880–1910

## Dissertations and Theses

Adirim, Genia. "Das medizinische Frauenstudium in Russland." Free University of Berlin, 1984.
Antler, Joyce. "The Educated Woman and Professionalization: The Struggle for New Feminine Identity, 1890–1920." State University of New York, Stony Brook, 1977.
Bachmann, Barbara, and Elke Bradenahl. "Medizinstudium von Frauen in Bern, 1871–1914." University of Bern, 1990.
Blumenthal, Annemarie. "Diskussionen um das medizinische Frauenstudium in Berlin." Free University of Berlin, 1965.
Burger, Elisabeth. "Die Entwicklung des medizinischen Frauenstudiums." University of Marburg, 1947.
Drachman, Virginia G. "Women Doctors and the Women's Medical Movement: Feminism and Medicine, 1850–1895." State University of New York, Buffalo, 1976.

Dudgeon, Ruth. "Women and Higher Education in Russia, 1855–1905." George Washington University, 1975.

Elston, Mary Ann C. "Women Doctors in the British Health Services: A Sociological Study of Their Careers and Opportunities." University of Leeds, 1986.

Fee, Elizabeth. "Science and the 'Woman Question,' 1860–1920: A Study of English Scientific Periodicals." Princeton University, 1978.

Foster, Pauline P. "Ann Preston, M.D. (1813–1872): A Biography. The Struggle to Obtain Training and Acceptance for Women Physicians in Mid-Nineteenth Century America." University of Pennsylvania, 1984.

Ganss, Erika. "Die Entwicklung des Frauenmedizinstudiums an deutschen Universitäten unter besonderer Berücksichtigung der Philipps-Universität in Marburg." University of Marburg, 1983.

Gilbert, Julie S. "Women at the English Civic Universities: 1880–1920." University of North Carolina, 1988.

Goldstein, Linda L. "Roses Bloomed in Winter: Women Medical Graduates of Western Reserve College, 1852–1856." Case Western Reserve University, 1989.

Hamilton, S. "Women and the Scottish Universities circa 1869–1939: A Social History." University of Edinburgh, 1987.

Hollmann, Raymond. "Die Stellungnahme der Ärzte im Streit um das Medizinstudium der Frau bis zum Beginn des 20. Jahrhunderts." University of Münster, 1976.

Luhn, Antke. "Geschichte des Frauenstudiums an der medizinischen Fakultät der Universität Göttingen." University of Göttingen, 1971.

Lutzker, Edythe. "Medical Education for Women in Great Britain." Columbia University, 1959.

Nahon, Roland. "Contribution à l'étude de l'accession des femmes à la carrière médicale à la fin du XIXᵉ siècle." University of Paris Val de Marne, 1978.

Pope, Rhama D. "The Development of Formal Higher Education for Women in England, 1862–1914." University of Pennsylvania, 1972.

Sahli, Nancy A. "Elizabeth Blackwell, M.D. (1821–1910): A Biography." University of Pennsylvania, 1974.

Tournier, Michèle. "L'accès des femmes aux études universitaires en France et en Allemagne (1861–1967)." University of Paris René Descartes, 1972.

Weisz, George. "La creation des universités françaises, 1885–1914." University of Paris V, 1980.

## Miscellaneous Unpublished Papers

Bickel, Janet. "Women in Medicine Statistics." Association of American Medical Colleges, May 1990.

Goldstein, Linda. "Without Compromise of Delicate Feeling." Paper delivered at the sixtieth meeting of the American Association for the History of Medicine, May 1987, Philadelphia.

Morantz-Sanchez, Regina M. "Women Physicians, Coeducation, and the Struggle for Professional Standards in Nineteenth-Century Medical Education." Paper presented at Berkshire Conference on the History of Women, August 1978.

Progin, Marianna, and Werner Seitz. "Das Frauenstudium an der Universitaet Bern." Historisches Seminar, University of Bern, 1980.

Saurer, J., and G. Beran. "Auslaendische Studieriende an der Universitaet Bern, 1834–1979." Historisches Seminar, University of Bern, [1980].


*Contemporary Books, Pamphlets, and Articles* (before 1918)

Agnew, D. Hayes. *Introductory Lecture to the One Hundred and Fifth Course of Instruction in the Medical Department of the University of Pennsylvania.* Philadelphia: R. P. King's Son, 1870.

Albert, E. *Die Frauen und das Studium der Medicin.* Vienna: Alfred Hölder, 1895.

Bennett, A. H. *English Medical Women: Glimpses of Their Work in Peace and War.* London: Isaac Pitman & Sons, 1915.

Benz, E., ed. *Die Frauenbewegung in der Schweiz.* Zurich: Th. Schröter, 1902.

Bert, Paul. "Les femmes et l'internat des hôpitaux." *Le Voltaire,* 1884.

Bischoff, Theodor L. W. von. *Das Studium und die Ausübung der Medicin durch Frauen.* Munich: Literarisch-Artistische Anstalt, 1872.

Blackwell, Elizabeth. *Address on the Medical Education of Women.* New York: Baptist and Taylor, 1864.

——— *Pioneer Work in Opening the Medical Profession to Women.* London: Longmans, Green, 1895.

Blackwell, Elizabeth, and Emily Blackwell. *Medicine as a Profession for Women.* New York: W. H. Tinson, 1860.

Bluhm, Agnes. "Die Entwicklung und der gegenwärtige Stand des medicinischen Frauenstudiums in den europäischen und aussereuropäischen Ländern." *Deutsche medicinische Wochenschrift,* 1895, *21:* 648–650.

Bodley, Rachel L. *Valedictory Address to the Twenty-Ninth Graduating Class of the Woman's Medical College of Pennsylvania.* Philadelphia: Grant, Faires & Rodgers, 1881.

Böhmert, Victor. *Das Frauenstudium nach den Erfahrungen an der Züricher Universität.* Leipzig, 1874.

——— *Rückblicke und Ausblicke eines Siebzigers.* Dresden: O. V. Böhmert, 1900.

——— *Das Studieren der Frauen mit besonderer Rücksicht auf das Studium der Medicin.* Leipzig: Otto Wigand, 1872.

——— *Das Studium der Frauen an der Universität Zürich.* Zurich, 1870.

——— *Die Zweite Doctorpromotion einer Dame in Zürich.* Zurich, 1870.

Bowditch, Henry I. "The Medical Education of Women." *Boston Medical and Surgical Journal,* 1879, *101:* 67–69.

——— "The Medical Education of Women. The Present Hostile Position of Harvard University and of the Massachusetts Medical Society. What Remedies Therefor Can Be Suggested?" *Boston Medical and Surgical Journal,* 1881, *105:* 289–293.

Bowditch, Vincent Y. *Life and Correspondence of Henry Ingersoll Bowditch.* Two volumes. Boston and New York: Houghton Mifflin, 1902.

Braun, Lily. *Die Frauenfrage: Ihre geschichtliche und wirtschaftliche Seite.* Leipzig: S. Hirzel, 1901.

Bridges, Flora. "Coeducation in Swiss Universities." *Popular Science Monthly,* 1891, *38:* 524–530.

Chadwick, James R. "The Study and Practice of Medicine by Women." *International Review,* October 1879, 444–471.

Clarke, Edward H. *Sex in Education; or, A Fair Chance for the Girls.* Boston: James R. Osgood, 1874.

Cohn, Gustav. "Die deutsche Frauenbewegung." *Deutsche Rundschau,* 1896, *86:* 404–432.

Cornell, William M. "The Medical Education of Women." *Boston Medical and Surgical Journal,* 1853, *49:* 419–422.

Dall, Caroline H., ed. *A Practical Illustration of "Woman's Right to Labor" or A Letter from Marie E. Zakrzewska, M.D., Late of Berlin, Prussia.* Boston: Walker, Wise, and Co., 1860.

Dimock, Susan. *Memoir of Susan Dimock.* Boston, 1875.

Erismann, Friedrich. *Gemeinsames Universitätsstudium für Männer und Frauen, oder besondere Frauen-Hochschulen.* Reprinted from *Die Frau,* 1899, 9–10.

——— "Khodataistva Pravleniia ob otkrytii vysshikh zhenskikh kursov i o pravakh zhenshchin vrachei, obuchaushikhsia zagranitsei." *Zhurnal obshchestva russkikh vrachei v pamiat N.I. Pirogova* (Moscow), 1895, *1:* 15–21.

——— "Das medizinische Studium und die ärztliche Praxis der Frauen." *Die Frau,* 1893–94, *1:* 747–749.

Eulenberg, A. "Das Medizinstudium der Frauen in den deutschen Universitäten im Sommersemester 1901." *Deutsche medizinische Wochenschrift,* 1901, *27:* 472.

Fehling, H. *Die Bestimmung der Frau: Ihre Stellung zu Familie und Beruf.* Stuttgart: Ferdinand Enke, 1892.

Female Medical College of Pennsylvania. *Announcement of a Course of Medical Lectures to Women in the City of Boston by the Faculty of the Female Medical College of Pennsylvania.* Boston, 1851.

Fickert, Auguste. "Das Medicinstudium der Frauen." *Wiener klinische Rundschau,* 1899, *13:* 241–243.

Figner, Vera. *Memoirs of a Revolutionist.* New York: International Publishers, 1927.

Flexner, Abraham. *Medical Education in Europe.* New York: Carnegie Foundation for the Advancement of Teaching, Bulletin no. 6, 1912.

——— *Medical Education in the United States and Canada.* New York: Carnegie Foundation for the Advancement of Teaching, Bulletin no. 4, 1910.

Fontanges, Haryett. *Les femmes docteurs en médecine des tous les pays.* 3rd ed. Paris: Alliance Coopérative du Livre, 1901.

Forster, Emily L. B. *How to Become a Woman Doctor.* London: Charles Griffin, 1918.

Girault, Augustine (pseud. A. Gaël). *La femme médecin: sa raison d'être au point de vue du droit, de la moralité et de l'humanité.* Paris: E. Dentu, 1868.

Goodell, William. *The Dangers and Duties of the Hour*. Baltimore: J. W. Borst, 1881.

Gregory, Samuel. *Letter to Ladies, in Favor of Female Physicians for Their Own Sex*. Boston: Female Medical Education Society, 1850.

Harrington, Thomas F. *The Harvard Medical School: A History, Narrative and Documentary*. Three volumes. New York: Lewis Publishing Company, 1905.

Henius, L. "Ueber die Zulassung der Frauen zum Studium der Medicin." *Deutsche medicinische Wochenschrift*, 1895, *21:* 613–615.

Henke, H. *Statistik der Universität Zürich in den ersten fünfzig Jahren ihres Bestehens von Ostern 1833 bis Ostern 1883*. Zurich: Zürcher and Furrer, 1883.

——— *Statistik der Universität Zürich von Ostern 1883 bis Ostern 1896*. Zurich: Zürcher and Furrer, 1896.

Henrich-Wilhelmi. *Das Recht der Frauen zum Studium und ihre Befähigung für alle Berufs-Arten*. Munich: Majer & Finch, [1894].

Hermann, Ludimar. *Erinnerungen*. Berlin, 1915.

——— *Das Frauenstudium und die Interessen der Hochschule Zürich*. Zurich, 1872.

Hunt, Harriot K. *Glances and Glimpses; or Fifty Years Social, Including Twenty Years Professional Life*. Boston: John P. Jewett, 1856.

International Congress of Women. *Women in Professions*. Two volumes. London: T. Fisher Unwin, 1900.

Jacobi, Abraham. "Das medicinische Frauenstudium in Amerika." *Deutsche medicinische Wochenschrift*, 1896, *22:* 401–403.

Jacobi, Mary Putnam. "Woman in Medicine." In *Woman's Work in America*, ed. Annie Nathan Meyer. New York: Henry Holt, 1891.

——— "Women in Medicine." In *What America Owes to Women*, ed. Lydia Hoyt Farmer. Buffalo: National Exposition Souvenir, 1893.

Jakoby, Hermann. *Grenzen der weiblichen Bildung*. Gütersloh: C. Bertelsmann, 1871.

Jex-Blake, Sophia. *Medical Women: A Thesis and a History*. Edinburgh: Oliphant, Anderson, & Ferrier, 1886.

——— *A Visit to Some American Schools and Colleges*. London: Macmillan, 1867.

Kirchoff, Arthur. *Die akademische Frau: Gutachten hervorragenden Universitätsprofessoren, Frauenlehrer und Schriftsteller uber die Befähigung der Frau zum wissenschaftlichen Studium und Berufe*. Berlin: Hugo Steinitz, 1897.

Kropotkin, Sophie. "The Higher Education of Women in Russia." *Nineteenth Century*, 1898, *43:* 117–134.

Lange, Helene. *Frauenbildung*. Berlin: L. Dehmigke's Verlag, 1889.

——— *Higher Education of Women in Europe*. New York: D. Appleton, 1890. Translated from German by L. R. Klemm.

Lange, Helene, and Gertrud Bäumer. *Handbuch der Frauenbewegung*. Four volumes. Berlin: W. Moeser, 1901.

Lassar, O. *Das medicinische Studium der Frau*. Berlin: S. Karger, 1897.

Lattin, Cora B. "The Woman Physician in Foreign Clinics." *Woman's Medical Journal*, 1910, *20:* 81–83.

Lipinska, Melanie. *Histoire des femmes médecins*. Paris: G. Jacques, 1900.

*London (Royal Free Hospital) School of Medicine for Women.* London, 1915.

London School of Medicine for Women. *Prospectus, 1886–87.* London, 1886.

—— *Report, 1890.* London, 1890.

MacMurchy, Helen. "Hospital Appointments. Are They Open to Women?" *New York Medical Journal,* 27 April 1901, 1–16.

Macy, Mary S. "Post-Graduate Medical Work for Women in Europe." *Woman's Medical Journal,* 1910, *20:* 59–61.

Madisson, Isabel. *Handbook of Courses Open to Women in British, Continental and Canadian Universities.* New York: Macmillan, 1896.

Malozemova, A. I. "Zhenshchiny-mediki v politicheskikh protsessakh 1881 g. (k. 100-letiiu protsessov)." *Sovetskoe zdravookhranenie,* 1881, *7:* 54–59.

Mann, Kristine. "Medical Women's Handicap," *Harper's Weekly,* 1914, *58:* 32.

Marshall, Clara. *The Woman's Medical College of Pennsylvania.* Philadelphia: P. Blakiston, 1897.

Ministère de l'Instruction Publique. *Bulletin administratif,* 1898–1914. Paris, 1899–1915.

Möbius, P. J. *Über den physiologischen Schwachsinn des Weibes.* Third edition. Halle: Carl Marhold, 1901.

Montanier, H. "La femme médecin." *Gazette des hôpitaux,* 1868, *34:* 1–2.

Neustätter, Otto. *Das Frauenstudium im Ausland.* Munich: August Schupp, 1899.

New England Hospital for Women and Children. *Marie Elizabeth Zakrzewska: A Memoir.* Boston, 1903.

Pagel, Julius. *Grundriss eines Systems der medizinischen Kulturgeschichte.* Berlin, 1905.

Penn Medical College of Philadelphia. *Announcement of the Penn Medical College of Philadelphia, Female Session.* Philadelphia: G. S. Harris, 1853.

Pope, Emily F., Emma L. Call, and C. Augusta Pope. *The Practice of Medicine by Women in the United States.* Boston: Wright & Potter, 1881.

Presbyterian Hospital and Woman's Medical College, Cincinnati. *Announcement, 1894–95.* Cincinnati, 1894.

Putnam, James J. "Women at Zurich." *Boston Medical and Surgical Journal,* 1879, *101:* 567–568.

Rabinowitsch, Lydia. "Die amerikanischen Frauen und ihre Leistungen." *Die Frauenbewegung,* 1897, *3:* 1–4.

Rose, Edmund. *Der Zürcher Hülfszug zum Schlachtfeld bei Belfort.* Zurich: Cäsar Schmidt, 1871.

Rosenfeld, Siegfried. "Das Medizinstudium der Frauen in der Gegenwart." *Wiener medizinische Blätter,* 1861, *19:* 6–9.

Scheel, H. von. *Frauenfrage und Frauenstudium: Rectoratsrede, Nov. 15, 1873.* Jena: Druck der Friedrich Mauke'schen Officen, 1873.

Scherr, Johannes. *Die Nihilisten.* Leipzig: Otto Wigand, 1885.

Schirmacher, Kaethe. *The Modern Woman's Rights Movement: A Historical Survey.* Second edition. New York: Macmillan, 1912.

—— *Züricher Studentinnen.* Zurich: Th. Schröter, 1896.

Schleinitz, Alexandra von. *Offener Brief einer Studirenden an die Gegner der ''Stu-*

*dentinnen''* *unter den Studenten und Berichtigung dieses Schreibens.* Zurich: Orell, Füssli, 1872.

Schubert-Feder, Cläre. *Das Leben der Studentinnen in Zürich.* Third edition. Berlin: R. Boll, 1894.

Schultze, Caroline. *La femme-médecin au XIX^e siècle.* Paris: Librairie Ollier-Henry, 1888.

Schwalbe, J. *Über das medizinische Frauenstudium in Deutschland.* Leipzig: Georg Thieme, 1918.

Sewall, May Wright, ed. *The World's Congress of Representative Women.* New York: Rand McNally, 1894.

Späth, Joseph. "Das Studium der Medizin und die Frauen." *Wiener medizinische Presse,* 1872, *13:* 1110–1118.

Stansfeld, James. "Medical Women." *Nineteenth Century,* 1877, *1:* 888–901.

Stanton, Theodore, ed. *The Woman Question in Europe.* New York: G. P. Putnam's Sons, 1884.

Sushchinskii, P. P. *Zhenshchina-vrach v Rossi: Ocherk desiatiletiia zhenskikh vrach-ebnykh kursov 1872–1882 god.* St. Petersburg, 1883.

Svatikov, Sergei. "Russkaii studentka: 1860–1915." In *Put'studenchestva* (Moscow, 1916), pp. 1–22.

Tait, Lawson. "The Medical Education of Women." *Birmingham Medical Review,* 1874, 81–94.

Teplov, Vasilii. "Piatidesiatiletie vysshago zhenskago obrazovaniia v Rossii." *Vestnik vospitaniia,* 1910, *9:* 117–132.

Thorne, Isabel. *Sketch of the Foundation and the Development of the London School of Medicine for Women.* London: G. Sharron, 1905.

Tiburtius, Franziska. "The Development of the Study of Medicine for Women in Germany, and Present Status." *Canadian Practitioner and Review,* 1909, *34:* 492–500.

———— "Frauenuniversitäten oder gemeinsames Studium?" *Die Frau,* 1898, *5:* 577–585.

U.S. Census Bureau. *A Compendium of the Ninth Census (June 1, 1870).* Washington: Government Printing Office, 1872.

———— *Compendium of the Tenth Census (June 1, 1880).* Two volumes. Washington: Government Printing Office, 1883.

U.S. Commissioner of Education. *Report for the Year 1870.* Washington: Government Printing Office, 1875.

Université de Genève. *Historique des Facultés, 1896–1914.* Geneva: Georg & Co., 1914.

Upham, Ella P. "Women in Medicine." *North American Journal of Homeopathy,* 1908, *56:* 341–348.

*Die Verläumdung der in Zürich studirenden russischen Frauen durch die russische Regierung.* Zurich: Druck der Genossenschafts-Buchdruckerei, [1873].

Wager, Mary A. E. "Women as Physicians." *Galaxy,* 1868, *6:* 774–789.

Waite, Frederick C. *History of the New England Female Medical College, 1848–1874.* Boston: Boston University School of Medicine, 1950.

Weber, Mathilde. *Ärztinnen für Frauenkrankheiten: Eine ethische und eine sanitäre Notwendigkeit.* Tübingen: Franz Fues, 1888.
——— *Ein Besuch in Zürich bei den weiblichen Studierenden der Medizin.* Stuttgart: W. Kohlhammer, 1888.
Woman's Medical College of Cincinnati. *Announcement, 1894–5.* Cincinnati, 1894.
Woman's Medical College of Georgia. *First Annual Announcement.* Atlanta: American Book and Job Print, 1889.
Woman's Medical College, Kansas City, Missouri. *First Annual Announcement.* Kansas City: Hudson-Kimberly, 1895.
Woman's Medical College of the New York Infirmary. *Final Catalogue.* [New York, 1899].
Woman's Medical College of Pennsylvania Alumnae Association. *Transactions of the Twenty-Fifth Annual Meeting.* Philadelphia, 1900.
Woman's Medical College, Toronto. *Seventh Annual Announcement, 1889–90.* Toronto: Brough & Caswell, 1889.
Woman's Medical College and Woman's Hospital of St. Louis. *Annual Announcement.* St. Louis, 1895.
Women's Medical Association of New York City. *In Memory of Dr. Elizabeth Blackwell and Dr. Emily Blackwell.* New York: Academy of Medicine, 1911.
Women's Medical College, Kingston. *Sixth Annual Calendar.* Kingston: British Whig Office, 1888.
Zakrzewska, Marie A. "Fifty Years Ago—A Retrospect." *Woman's Medical Journal,* 1893, *1:* 193–195.
Zehender, Wilhelm von. *Ueber den Beruf der Frauen zum Studium und zur praktischen Ausbildung der Heilwissenschaft.* Rostock: Stiller'sche Hof- und Universitätsbuchhandlung, 1875.

*Books and Articles Since 1918*

Abrahams, Harold J. *The Extinct Medical Schools of Baltimore, Maryland.* Baltimore: Maryland Historical Society, 1969.
——— *Extinct Medical Schools of Nineteenth-Century Philadelphia.* Philadelphia: University of Pennsylvania Press, 1966.
Abram, Ruth J., ed. *"Send Us a Lady Physician": Women Doctors in America, 1835–1920.* New York: W. W. Norton, 1985.
Albisetti, James C. "Could Separate Be Equal? Helene Lange and Women's Education in Imperial Germany." *History of Education Quarterly,* 1982, *22:* 301–317.
——— "The Fight for Female Physicians in Imperial Germany." *Central European History,* 1982, *15:* 99–123.
——— *Schooling German Girls and Women: Secondary and Higher Education in the Nineteenth Century.* Princeton: Princeton University Press, 1988.
——— "Women and the Professions in Imperial Germany." In *German Women in the Eighteenth and Nineteenth Centuries: A Social and Literary History,* ed.

Ruth-Ellen B. Joeres and Mary Jo Maynes. Bloomington: Indiana University Press, 1986.

Alexander, Wendy. *First Ladies of Medicine: The Origins, Education and Destination of Early Women Medical Graduates of Glasgow University.* Glasgow: Wellcome Unit for the History of Medicine, 1988.

Alsop, Gulielma F. *History of the Woman's Medical College, Philadelphia, Pennsylvania.* Philadelphia: J. B. Lippincott, 1950.

American Public Health Association. *Women in Health Careers: Chart Book for International Conference on Women in Health Held at Washington, D.C., on June 16–18, 1975.* Washington: Health Resources Administration, 1975.

Anderson, Louisa Garrett. *Elizabeth Garrett Anderson, 1836–1917.* London: Faber and Faber, [1939].

Anderson, R. D. *Education and Opportunity in Victorian Scotland.* Oxford: Clarendon Press, 1983.

André-Thomas. "Augusta Déjerine-Klumpke, 1859–1927." *L'Encephale,* 1928, 75–88.

*Annuaire statistique de la France, 1920–1967.* Paris, 1921–1968.

Aptheker, Bettina. *Woman's Legacy: Essays on Race, Sex, and Class in American History.* Amherst: University of Massachusetts Press, 1982.

Bankowski-Züllig, Monika. "Russischer Alltag im Plattenquartier." *Uni Zürich,* April, 1986, 10–12.

Barlow, William, and David O. Powell. "A Case for Medical Coeducation in the 1870s." *Journal of the American Medical Women's Association,* 1980, *35:* 285–288.

Bazanov, V. A. "Nadezhda Suslova—pervaia russkaia zhenshchina-vrach." *Feld'sher i akusherka* (Moscow), 1963, *9:* 51–55.

Bell, E. Moberly. *Storming the Citadel: The Rise of the Woman Doctor.* London: Constable, 1953.

Bernier, J.-J. "Croissance du corps médical." *Nouvelle presse médicale,* 1976, *5:* 517–519.

Bleker, Johanna, and Heinz-Peter Schmiedebach, eds. *Medizin und Krieg: vom Dilemma der Heilberufe, 1865 bis 1915.* Fischer Taschenbuch, [1985].

Blochmann, Maria. *Lass dich gelüsten nach der Männer Weisheit und Bildung.* Pfaffenweiler: Centaurus, 1990.

Boehm, Laetitia. "Von den Anfängen des akademischen Frauenstudiums in Deutschland: Zugleich ein Kapitel aus der Geschichte der Ludwig-Maximilians-Universität München." *Historisches Jahrbuch,* 1958, *77:* 298–327.

Bonner, Thomas N. *American Doctors and German Universities: A Chapter in International Intellectual Relations.* Lincoln: University of Nebraska Press, Landmark Edition, 1988.

——— *Medicine in Chicago, 1850–1950: A Chapter in the Social and Scientific Development of a City.* Second edition. Urbana: University of Illinois Press, 1991.

Borgeaud, Charles, ed. *Histoire de l'Université de Genève.* Four volumes. Geneva: Georg & Co., 1934.

Bourdillon, Hilary. *Women as Healers: A History of Women and Medicine.* Cambridge: Cambridge University Press, 1988.

Bowers, John Z. "Women in Medicine: An International Study." *New England Journal of Medicine,* 1966, *275:* 362–365.

Brentjes, Sonja, and Karl-Heinz Schlote. "Zum Frauenstudium an der Universität Leipzig in der Zeit von 1870 bis 1910." *Perspektiven interkultureller Wechselwirkung für den wissenschaftlichen Fortschritt,* Akademie der Wissenschaften der DDR Kolloquien, 1985, *48:* 21–29.

Burstyn, Joan N. "Education and Sex: The Medical Case against Higher Education for Women in England, 1870–1900." *Proceedings of the American Philosophical Society,* 1973, *117:* 78–89.

————— *Victorian Education and the Ideal of Womanhood.* London: Croom Helm, 1980.

Butcher, Patricia S. *Education for Equality: Women's Rights Periodicals and Women's Higher Education, 1849–1920.* Westport, Conn.: Greenwood Press, 1989.

Calmes, Selma H. "Rose Talbot Bullard MD: LACMA's Only Woman President." *Los Angeles County Medical Association Physician,* 17 October 1983, pp. 26–28.

Chesney, Alan M. *The Johns Hopkins Hospital and the Johns Hopkins University School of Medicine.* Three volumes. Baltimore: Johns Hopkins Press, 1943–1963.

Cole, Stephen. "Sex Discrimination and Admission to Medical School, 1929–1984." *American Journal of Sociology,* 1986, *92:* 549–555.

Craig, Gordon A. *The Germans.* New York: New American Library, 1982.

————— *The Triumph of Liberalism: Zürich in the Golden Age, 1830–1869.* New York: Scribner's, 1988.

Cramer, Marc, and Jean Starobinski. *Centenaire de la faculté de médecine de l'Université de Genève (1876–1976): Documents.* Geneva: Editions Médecine et Hygiène, 1978.

Dionesov, Semen M. "Russkie tsiurikhskie studentkimedichki v revoliutsionnom dvizhenii 70-kh godov xix stoletiia." *Sovetskoe zdravookhranenie,* 1973, *11:* 68–72.

————— *V. A. Kashevarova-Rudneva—pervia russkaia zhenshchina-doktor meditsiny.* Moscow, 1965.

Dobkin, Marjorie H. *The Making of a Feminist: Early Journals and Letters of M. Carey Thomas.* Kent, Ohio: Kent State University Press, 1979.

Drachman, Virginia. *Hospital with a Heart: Women Doctors and the Paradox of Separatism at the New England Hospital, 1862–1969.* Ithaca: Cornell University Press, 1984.

————— "The Limits of Progress: The Professional Lives of Women Doctors, 1881–1926." *Bulletin of the History of Medicine,* 1986, *60:* 58–72.

Drucker, Renate. "Zur Vorgeschichte des Frauenstudiums an der Universität Leipzig." In *Vom Mittelalter zur Neuzeit,* ed. Hellmut Kretzschmar, pp. 278–282. Berlin: Rütten & Loening, 1956.

Dudgeon, Ruth. "The Forgotten Minority: Women Students in Imperial Russia, 1872–1917." *Russian History/Histoire Russe,* 1982, *9:* 1–26.

Duruy, Victor. "Une conquête du feminisme sous le Second Empire: Fondation d'une école pour l'instruction médicale des femmes." *Bulletin de l'enseignement public au Moroc*, 1954, *229:* 51–61.

Dutkowa, Renata. "Les études de jeunes Polonais dans les universités étrangères au XIXᵉ siècle." In *Peregrinations academiques*. Cracow: Nakładem Uniwersytetu Jagiellońskiego, 1989.

Dykman, Roscoe A., and John M. Stalnaker. "Survey of Women Physicians Graduating from Medical School, 1925–1940." *Journal of Medical Education*, 1957, *32:* 3–35.

Eidgenössisches Statistisches Amt. *Schweizerische Hochschulstatistik, 1890–1935.* Bern, 1935.

Elston, Mary Ann. "Women's Access to Medical Education in Great Britain, 1877–1900: An Overview." *Bulletin of the Society for the Social History of Medicine*, 1987, *41:* 51–53.

Engel, Barbara A. "Women Medical Students in Russia, 1872–1882: Reformers or Rebels?" *Journal of Social History*, 1978, *12:* 394–414.

Engel, Barbara A., and Clifford N. Rosenthal, eds. *Five Sisters: Women against the Tsar.* Boston: Allen & Unwin, 1987.

Erb, Hans. *Geschichte der Studentenschaft an der Universität Zurich, 1833–1936.* Zurich: Müller, Werder, 1937.

Evans, Richard J. *The Feminist Movement in Germany, 1894–1933.* London: Sage Publications, 1976.

Evans, Sara M. *Born for Liberty: A History of Women in America.* New York: Free Press, 1989.

Fee, Elizabeth. "Nineteenth-Century Craniology: The Study of the Female Skull." *Bulletin of the History of Medicine*, 1979, *53:* 415–433.

Feller, Richard. *Die Universität Bern 1834–1934.* Bern: Paul Haupt, 1935.

Filar, Zbigniew. *Anna Tomaszewicz Dobrska: A Leaf from Polish Medical History.* Warsaw: Polish Society of the History of Medicine, 1959.

Forel, August. *Briefe: Correspondance, 1864–1927.* Bern: Hans Huber, 1968.

——— *Out of My Life and Work.* New York: W. W. Norton, 1937.

——— *Rückblick auf mein Leben.* Zurich: Europa-Verlag, 1934.

Forkl, Martha, and Elisabeth Koffmann, eds. *Frauenstudium und akademische Frauenarbeit in Österreich.* Vienna, 1968.

Frieden, Nancy M. *Russian Physicians in an Era of Reform and Revolution, 1856–1905.* Princeton: Princeton University Press, 1981.

Gagliardi, Ernst, Hans Nabholz, and Jean Strohl. *Die Universität Zürich 1833–1933: Festschrift zur Jahrhundertfeier.* Zurich: Erziehungsdirektion, 1938

Galenson, Marjorie. *Women and Work: An International Comparison.* Ithaca: New York State School of Industrial and Labor Relations, 1973.

Gerber, John C. *A Pictorial History of the University of Iowa.* Iowa City: University of Iowa Press, 1988.

Geyer-Kordesch, Johanna. "Geschlecht und Gesellschaft: Die ersten Ärztinnen und sozialpolitische Vorurteile." *Berichte zur Wissenschaftsgeschichte*, 1987, *10:* 195–205.

Gordon, Lynn D. *Gender and Higher Education in the Progressive Era.* New Haven: Yale University Press, 1990.

Green, Nancy. "L'émigration comme émancipation: les femmes juives d'Europe de l'est à Paris, 1881–1914." *Pluriel de bat*, 1981, *27:* 51–59.

Guggisberg, Hans R. "Eine Amerikanerin in Zürich: Die Doktorpromotion der Martha Carey Thomas aus Baltimore (1882)." In *Zürcher Taschenbuch 1982.* Zurich: Buchdruckerei an der Sihl, 1981.

Hacker, Carlotta. *The Indomitable Lady Doctors.* Toronto: Clarke, Irwin, 1974.

Hamilton, Alice. *Exploring the Dangerous Trades: The Autobiography of Alice Hamilton, M.D.* Boston: Little, Brown, 1943.

Hausen, Karin, and Helga Nowotny, eds. *Wie männlich ist die Wissenschaft?* Frankfurt am Main: Suhrkamp, 1986.

Hellstedt, Leone M., ed. *Women Physicians of the World.* Washington: Hemisphere Publishing Co., 1978.

Hildreth, Martha L. "Delicacy and Propriety: The Acceptance of the Woman Physician in Victorian America." *Halcyon*, 1987, *9:* 149–165.

Hofstätter, R. "Über das Hochschulstudium der Frauen in Österreich mit besonderer Berücksichtigung des ärztlichen Berufes." *Archiv für Frauenkunde und Konstitutions Forschung*, 1929, *16:* 301–319.

Hurd-Mead, Kate C. *Medical Women of America: A Short History of the Pioneer Medical Women of America and of a Few of Their Colleagues in England.* New York: Froben Press, 1933.

Hyde, Ida H. "Before Women Were Human Beings . . . Adventures of an American Fellow in German Universities of the '90s." *Journal of the American Association of University Women*, 1937–1939, *31–32:* 226–236.

James, Edward T., and Janet W. James, eds. *Notable American Women.* Three volumes. Cambridge, Mass.: Belknap Press of Harvard University Press, 1971.

Jarausch, Konrad H. *Students, Society, and Politics in Imperial Germany: The Rise of Academic Illiberalism.* Princeton: Princeton University Press, 1982.

Jewsbury, George. "Russian Students in Nancy, France: 1905–1914. A Case Study." *Jahrbücher für Geschichte Osteuropas*, 1975, *23:* 225–228.

Joël, Constance. *Les filles d'Esculape: Les femmes à la conquête du pouvoir médical.* Paris: Robert Laffont, 1988.

Johanson, Christine. "Autocratic Politics, Public Opinion, and Women's Medical Education during the Reign of Alexander II, 1855–1881." *Slavic Review*, 1979, *38:* 426–443.

———— *Women's Struggle for Higher Education in Russia, 1855–1900.* Kingston and Montreal: McGill-Queen's University Press, 1987.

Junginger, Gabriele, ed. *Maria Gräfin von Linden: Erinnerungen der ersten Tübinger Studentin.* Tübingen: Attempto, 1991.

Justin, Meryl S. "The Entry of Women into Medicine in America: Education and Obstacles, 1847–1910." *Synthesis*, 1978, *4:* 31–46.

Kaiser, Robert M., Sandra L. Chaff, and Steven J. Peitzman. "A Philadelphia Medical Student of the 1890's: The Diary of Mary Theodora McGavran." *Pennsylvania Magazine of History and Biography*, 1984, *108:* 217–236.

Kater, Michael. *Doctors under Hitler.* Chapel Hill: University of North Carolina Press, 1989.

Kaufman, Martin, Stuart Galishoff, and Todd L. Savitt, eds. *Dictionary of American*

*Medical Biography.* Two volumes. Westport, Conn.: Greenwood Press, 1984.

Kelly, Paige. "Upstarts: Opposition Greeted First Women Medical Students." *Advance* (University of Michigan School of Medicine), summer 1982, 1–6.

Koblitz, Ann Hibner. *A Convergence of Lives: Sofia Kovalevskaia, Scientist, Writer, Revolutionary.* Boston: Birkhauser, 1983.

———— "Science, Women, and the Russian Intelligentsia: The Generation of the 1860s." *Isis,* 1988, *79:* 208–226.

"The Lady Doctor: What Barriers Does She Meet?" *Modern Medicine,* 21 October 1968, 54–64.

Leavitt, Judith W., ed. *Women and Health in America.* Madison: University of Wisconsin Press, 1984.

Lequay, Françoise, and Claude Barbizet. *Blanche Edwards-Pilliet: Femme et médecin 1858–1941.* LeMans: Editions Cénomane, 1988.

Lipinska, Mélanie. *Les femmes et le progrès des sciences médicales.* Paris: Masson, 1930.

Little, F. Graham. "Undergraduate Medical Education of Women in London." *Nineteenth Century,* 1928, 665–677.

Lopate, Carol. *Women in Medicine.* Baltimore: Johns Hopkins Press, 1968.

Lovejoy, Esther P. *Women Doctors of the World.* New York: Macmillan, 1957.

Lowther, Florence D., and Helen R. Downes. "Women in Medicine." *Journal of the American Medical Women's Association,* 1945, *129:* 512–514.

Ludmerer, Kenneth. *Learning to Heal: The Development of American Medical Education.* New York: Basic Books, 1985.

Lutzker, Edythe. *Women Gain a Place in Medicine.* New York: McGraw-Hill, 1969.

MacDermot, H. E. *Maude Abbott: A Memoir.* Toronto: Macmillan, 1941.

Macfarlane, Catharine. "The Woman's Medical College of Pennsylvania." *Transactions and Studies of the College of Physicians and Surgeons of Philadelphia,* 1965, *33:* 39–42.

Manton, Jo. *Elizabeth Garrett Anderson.* New York: E. P. Dutton, 1965.

Martindale, L. *A Woman Surgeon.* London: Victor Gollancz, 1951.

McGuigan, Dorothy G. *A Dangerous Experiment: 100 Years of Women at the University of Michigan.* Ann Arbor: Center for Continuing Education for Women, 1970.

Meijer, J. M. *Knowledge and Revolution: The Russian Colony in Zürich (1870–1873).* Assen, Netherlands: Van Gorcum, 1955.

Moldow, Gloria. *Women Doctors in Gilded-Age Washington.* Urbana: University of Illinois Press, 1987.

Morantz-Sanchez, Regina M. *Sympathy and Science: Women Physicians in American Medicine.* New York: Oxford University Press, 1985.

More, Ellen. "The Blackwell Medical Society and the Professionalization of Women Physicians." *Bulletin of the History of Medicine,* 1987, *61:* 603–628.

———— " 'A Certain Restless Ambition': Women Physicians and World War I." *American Quarterly,* 1989, *41:* 636–660.

Morgan, Beverly C. "Admission of Women into Medical Schools in the United States: Current Status." *Woman Physician,* 1971, *26:* 305–309.

Mysyrowicz, Ladislas. "Les étudiants 'orientaux' en médecine à Genève," *Gesnerus*, 1977, *34:* 207–212.

———. "Université et Révolution: Les étudiants d'Europe Orientale à Genève au temps de Plékhanov et de Lénine." *Revue suisse d'histoire*, 1975, *25:* 514–562.

Nauck, E. Th. *Das Frauenstudium an der Universität Freiburg I.Br.* Freiburg: Eberhard Albert Universitätsbuchhandlung, 1953.

Nekrasova, E. S. "Zhenskie vrachebnye kursy v Peterburge." *Vestnik Evropy*, 1982, *6:* 807–845.

Neumann, Daniela. *Studentinnen aus dem Russischen Reich in der Schweiz (1867–1914).* Zurich: Hans Rohr, 1987.

Odier-Dollfus. "Status of Medical Women in France." *Journal of the American Medical Women's Association*, 1948, *3:* 413–414.

Panteleev, L. F. *Vospominaniia.* Moscow, 1958.

Pavluchkova, A. V. "Bor'ba progressivnoi meditsinskoi obshchestvennosti za vvedenie zhenskogo vrachebnogo obrazovaniia v Rosii (60-e-nachalo 70 kh godov xix veka)." *Sovetskoe zdravookhranenia*, 1976, *4:* 58–62.

Peitzman, Steven J. "The Quiet Life of a Philadelphia Medical Woman: Mary Willits (1855–1902)." *Journal of the American Medical Women's Association*, 1979, *34:* 443–460.

Percebois, Gilbert. "Les femmes à la conquête de la médecine." *Annales médicales de Nancy*, 1977, 1259–1274.

Persons, Stow. "The Decline of Homeopathy—The University of Iowa, 1876–1919," *Bulletin of the History of Medicine*, 1991, *65:* 74–87.

Plaschka, Richard, and Karlheinz Mack, eds. *Wegenetz europäischen Geistes: Wissenschaftszentren und geistige wechselbeziehungen zwischen Mittel-und Südosteuropa vom Ende des 18. Jahrhunderts bis zum ersten Weltkrieg.* Munich: R. Oldenbourg, 1983.

———. *Wegenetz europäischen Geistes II: Universitäten und Studenten.* Munich: R. Oldenbourg, 1987.

Portmann, Marie-Louise. "Neue Aspekte zur Biographie des Basler Biochemikers Gustav von Bunge (1844–1920) aus seinem handschriftlichen Nachlass." *Gesnerus*, 1974, *31:* 39–46.

Puckett, Hugh W. *Germany's Women Go Forward.* New York: Columbia University Press, 1930.

Putnam, Ruth, ed. *Life and Letters of Mary Putnam Jacobi.* New York: G. P. Putnam's Sons, 1925.

Ringer, Fritz K. *Education and Society in Modern Europe.* Bloomington: Indiana University Press, 1979.

Robb-Smith, A. H. T. "The Fate of Oxford Medical Women." *Lancet*, 1 December 1962, 1158–1161.

Rohner, Hanny. *Die ersten 30 Jahre des medizinischen Frauenstudiums an der Universität Zürich 1867–1897.* Zurich: Juris Druck & Verlag, 1972.

Romieu, Claude. "Agnes McLaren, première femme docteur en médecine de la Faculté de Montpellier." *Monspeliensis Hippocrates*, 1966, *31:* 21–28.

Rosenberg, Carroll Smith, and Charles Rosenberg. "The Female Animal: Medical and Biological Views of Woman and Her Role in Nineteenth-Century America." *Journal of American History,* 1973, *60:* 332–356.

Rossiter, Margaret W. *Women Scientists in America: Struggles and Strategies to 1940.* Baltimore: Johns Hopkins University Press, 1982.

Rudd, Helga M. "The Women's Medical College of Chicago." *Medical Woman's Journal,* 1946, *53:* 41–46, 64.

Rupp, Elke. *Der Beginn des Frauenstudiums an der Universität Tübingen.* Tübingen: Universitätsarchiv, 1978.

Russett, Cynthia E. *Sexual Science: The Victorian Construction of Womanhood.* Cambridge, Mass.: Harvard University Press, 1989.

Ryan, Michael. *Doctors and the State in the Soviet Union.* New York: St. Martin's Press, 1990.

Ryten, Eva. "A Brief Statistical History of the Enrollment of Women in Medicine in Canada." *Nova Scotia Medical Journal,* February 1990, 15–18.

Sablik, K. "Zum Beginn des Frauenstudiums an der Wiener medizinischen Fakultät." *Wiener medizinische Wochenschrift,* 1968, *118:* 817–819.

St. John, Christopher. *Christine Murrell, M.D.: Her Life and Her Work.* London: Williams & Norgate, 1935.

Satran, Richard. "Augusta Déjerine-Klumpke: First Woman Intern in Paris Hospitals." *Annals of Internal Medicine,* 1974, *80:* 260–264.

Scandola, Pietro. *Hochschulgeschichte Berns 1528–1984.* Bern: Universität Bern, 1984.

Schönfeld, Walther. "Die Einstellung der Heidelberger medizinischen Fakultät in den achtziger Jahren zum Medizinstudium der Frauen." *Rupert-Carola,* 1961, *29:* 198–205.

———— *Frauen in der abendländischen Heilkunde: von klassischem Altertum bis zum Ausgang des 19. Jahrhunderts.* Stuttgart: Ferdinand Enke, 1947.

Schweizerischer Verband der Akademikerinnen. *Das Frauenstudium an den schweizer Hochschulen.* Zurich: Rascher, 1928.

Schwöbel-Schrafl, Eliane. *Was verdankt die medizinische Fakultät Zürich ihren ausländischen Dozenten? 1833 bis 1863.* Zurich: Juris Druck & Verlag, 1985.

Semashko, N. A. "Friedrich Erismann: The Dawn of Russian Hygiene and Public Health." *Bulletin of the History of Medicine,* 1946, *20:* 1–9.

Senn, Alfred E. *The Russian Revolution in Switzerland, 1914–1917.* Madison: University of Wisconsin Press, 1971.

Shaw, Wilfred B., ed. *The University of Michigan: An Encyclopedic Survey.* Four volumes. Ann Arbor: University of Michigan Press, 1951.

Shepherd, Nan. "Women in the University Fifty Years: 1892–1942." *Aberdeen University Review,* 1941–42, *29:* 171–181.

Shikes, Robert H., and Henry N. Claman. *The University of Colorado School of Medicine: A Centennial History, 1883–1983.* Denver: Board of Regents of the University of Colorado, 1983.

Shryock, Richard H. "Women in American Medicine." *Journal of the American Medical Women's Association,* 1950, *5:* 371–379.

Sicherman, Barbara. *Alice Hamilton: A Life in Letters.* Cambridge, Mass.: Harvard University Press, 1984.

Siebel, Johanna. *Das Leben von Frau Dr. Marie Heim-Vögtlin 1845–1916.* Zurich: Rascher, 1928.

Smith, Elizabeth. *"A Woman with a Purpose": The Diaries of Elizabeth Smith, 1872–1884.* Ed. Veronica Strong-Boag. Toronto: University of Toronto Press, 1980.

Solomon, Barbara. *In the Company of Educated Women: A History of Women and Higher Education in America.* New Haven: Yale University Press, 1985.

Steudel, Johannes. "Heilkundige Frauen des Abendlandes." *Zentralblatt für Gynäkologie,* 1959, *81:* 284–295.

Stites, Richard. *The Women's Liberation Movement in Russia: Feminism, Nihilism, and Bolshevism, 1860–1930.* Princeton: Princeton University Press, 1978.

Strachey, Ray. *"The Cause": A Short History of the Women's Movement in Great Britain.* Port Washington, N.Y.: Kennikat Press, 1969.

Strecker, Gabriele. "Medical Women in Germany." *Journal of the American Medical Women's Association,* 1947, *2:* 506–508.

Thelander, Hulda E., and Helen B. Weyrauch. "Women in Medicine." Reprinted from *Journal of the American Medical Association,* 1952, *148:* 1–11.

Thomas, Onfel. *Frances Elizabeth Hoggan, 1843–1927.* Privately printed, [1970].

Tiburtius, Franziska. *Erinnerungen einer Achtzigjährigen.* Third edition. Berlin: C. A. Schwetschke & Sohn, 1929.

Todd, Margaret. *The Life of Sophia Jex-Blake.* London: Macmillan, 1918.

Tracy, Martha. "Women Graduates in Medicine." *Association of American Medical Colleges Bulletin,* 1927, *2:* 21–28.

Truax, Rhoda. *The Doctors Jacobi.* Boston: Little, Brown, 1952.

Turner, A. Logan. *History of the University of Edinburgh, 1883–1933.* Edinburgh: Oliver and Boyd, 1933.

Tuve, Jeanette E. *The First Russian Women Physicians.* Newtonville, Mass.: Oriental Research Partners, 1984.

Tylecote, Mabel. *The Education of Women at Manchester University, 1833 to 1933.* Manchester: University of Manchester Press, 1941.

Université de Lausanne. *Cinquantenaire de la Faculté de Médecine de Lausanne 1890–1940.* Lausanne: F. Roth, [1940].

Van Hoosen, Bertha. *Petticoat Surgeon.* Chicago: Pellegrini & Cudahy, 1947.

Verbrugge, Martha H. "Women and Medicine in Nineteenth-Century America." *Signs,* 1976, *1:* 957–972.

Verein Feministische Wissenschaft Schweiz. *Ebenso neu als kühn: 120 Jahre Frauenstudium an der Universität Zürich.* Zurich, 1988.

Vietor, Agnes C., ed. *A Woman's Quest: The Life of Marie E. Zakrzewska, M.D.* New York: W. W. Norton, 1924.

Waite, Frederick C. "Medical Education of Women in Cleveland (1850–1930)." *Western Reserve Bulletin,* 1930, *16:* 1–29.

Walsh, Mary R. *"Doctors Wanted: No Women Need Apply": Sexual Barriers in the Medical Profession, 1835–1975.* New Haven: Yale University Press, 1977.

Warner, Deborah J. "Science Education for Women in Antebellum America." *Isis*, 1978, *69:* 58–67.

Weber, Marianne. *Frauenfragen und Frauengedanken: Gesammelte Aufsätze.* Tübingen: J. C. B. Mohr, 1919.

Weill, Claudie. "Les étudiants russes en Allemagne 1900–1914." *Cahiers du monde russe et sovietique,* 1979, *20:* 203–225.

Weisz, George. *The Emergence of Modern Universities in France, 1863–1914.* Princeton: Princeton University Press, 1983.

Weizmann, Chaim. *Trial and Error: The Autobiography of Chaim Weizmann.* New York: Harper, 1949.

Weizmann, Vera. *The Impossible Takes Longer.* London: Hamish Hamilton, 1967.

Whittaker, Cynthia H. "The Women's Movement during the Reign of Alexander II: A Case Study in Russian Liberalism." *Journal of Modern History,* 1976, *48:* 35–69 (on demand supplement).

Wick, Hanspeter. *Friedrich Huldreich Erismann (1842–1915): Russischer Hygieniker-Zürcher Stadtrat.* Zurich: Zürcher medizingeschichtliche Abhandlungen, new series no. 82, 1970.

Wolchik, Sharon L., and Alfred G. Meyer, eds. *Women, State, and Party in Eastern Europe.* Durham: Duke University Press, 1985.

Women's Medical Association of New York City, ed. *Mary Putnam Jacobi, M.D.: A Pathfinder in Medicine.* New York: G. P. Putnam's Sons, 1925.

Woodtli, Susanna. *Gleichberechtigung: Der Kampf um die politische Rechte der Frau in der Schweiz.* Frauenfeld: Huber, 1975.

Woody, Thomas. *A History of Women's Education in the United States.* Two volumes. New York: Science Press, 1929.

Zimmermann, Werner G., ed. *Schweiz-Russland: Begleitband zur Ausstellung der Präsidialabteilung der Stadt Zürich.* Zurich: Strauhof Zürich, 1989.

Zott, Regine. "Zu den Anfängen des Frauenstudiums an der Berliner Universität." *Perspektiven interkultureller Wechselwirkung für den wissenschaftlichen Fortschritt,* Akademie der Wissenschaften der DDR Kolloquien, 1985, *48:* 29–37.

# Index